The Mystery of
THE EXPLODING TEETH

THE MYSTERY OF

the

EXPLODING TEETH

And Other Curiosities from the History of Medicine

THOMAS MORRIS

DUTTON

DUTTON

An imprint of Penguin Random House LLC
penguinrandomhouse.com

Illustrations: page 129 reproduced courtesy of the US Patent Office; page 130 reproduced
courtesy of *Scientific American*; pages 145 and 148 reproduced courtesy of the Bodleian Library,
University of Oxford, 4° Z 46 Med., frontispiece and title. All other illustrations reproduced
courtesy of the Wellcome Libraries.

LIBRARY OF CONGRESS CATALOGING-IN-PUBLICATION DATA

Names: Morris, Thomas (Thomas Neil Gareth), author.
Title: The mystery of the exploding teeth : and other curiosities
from the history of medicine / Thomas Morris.
Description: New York, New York : Dutton, [2018] | Includes
bibliographical references and index.
Identifiers: LCCN 2018022919 | ISBN 9781524743680 (hardback) |
ISBN 9781524743697 (ebook)
Subjects: | MESH: Folklore | History of Medicine | Anecdotes
Classification: LCC R733 | NLM WZ 308 | DDC 610—dc23
LC record available at https://lccn.loc.gov/2018022919

Printed in the United States of America
1   3   5   7   9   10   8   6   4   2

BOOK DESIGN BY KATY RIEGEL

For Jenny

✳

CONTENTS

4. HORRIFYING OPERATIONS

*The case of the drunken Dutchman's guts * If you can't find a surgeon . . . * The self-inflicted lithotripsy * A high pain threshold * A window in his chest * The sad case of Hoo Loo * All at sea * An extraordinary surgical operation*

5. REMARKABLE RECOVERIES

*The wandering musket ball * The miller's tale * In one side and out the other * A bayonet through the head * An interesting and remarkable accident * The lucky Prussian * A case for Dr. Coffin * The healing power of nature * Severed, replaced, reunited * Give that man a medal * A bit of a headache*

6. TALL TALES

*Sleeping with the fishes * Death of a 152-year-old * The combustible countess * He sliced his penis in two * Half man, half snake * The human waxwork * The slugs and the porcupine * The amphibious infant * The seventy-year-old mother-to-be*

7. HIDDEN DANGERS

*A surfeit of cucumbers * The perils of being a writer * Why children should never wear hats * Killed by his false teeth * Pegged out * The cast-iron stove panic * Brolly painful * A flaming nuisance * Cycling will give you heart disease*

INTRODUCTION

A COUPLE OF YEARS ago I was sitting in a library, plowing through a rather dull nineteenth-century article about heart disease, when I spotted something more interesting on the previous page of the journal I was perusing. Underneath the promising headline "Sudden Protrusion of the whole of the Intestines into the Scrotum," I found the following:

> *John Marsh, aged 50, a labourer, was brought into the hospital, having just been run over by a cart laden with bricks. His scrotum, on inspection, was found to be of most enormous size, extending two thirds downwards between the thighs, and measuring in circumference 17 inches. Its colour of a jet black; and its texture, from over distention, so exquisitely thin as to threaten immediate rupture from the slightest manipulation.*

Questions whirled through my mind. Why was his scrotum so enormous? What on earth could a doctor do about such an injury in 1829? How long did the unfortunate John Marsh survive?

Horrified and fascinated in equal measure, I could not stop reading. The answers proved to be just as intriguing. When the cartwheels had passed over Mr. Marsh's belly, they had done so with such force that his intestines were squeezed through the inguinal canal, a narrow passage between the abdominal cavity and the scrotum. With his guts now competing with his nuts for scrotum space, as it were, the physicians had a simple task: Get them back where they belonged.

> *On being placed in bed the viscera were returned to their natural situation without much difficulty, merely by elevating the hips, depressing the shoulders, and applying moderate and careful pressure with flannels moistened in hot poppy fomentation.*

Hot-water bottles, laxatives, opium and leeches (applied to the scrotum) completed the treatment. My assumption about Mr. Marsh's survival prospects turned out to be unduly pessimistic.

> *On the twelfth day from the occurrence of the injury the patient was reported as quite convalescent, and able to sit up for some hours in bed, the precaution of applying a truss having previously been taken. At the end of the third week he was discharged cured.*

Not *quite* cured, it turned out. A postscript adds:

> *He is compelled to wear his double truss both night and day, otherwise the viscera descend immediately into the scrotum in very large quantities.*

I soon discovered that you can hardly flick through the pages of an old medical journal without stumbling across a story that is compellingly disgusting, hilarious or downright bizarre. In between long, dry dissertations on London sanitation or the treatment of yellow fever are scattered little anecdotal gems: tales of patients who glowed in the dark, performed surgery on their own bodies or vomited living slugs. Some are poignant or touching, a few are grim, but they all have more to offer than just a good yarn. However embarrassing the ailment or odd the treatment, every one of these cases says something about the beliefs and knowledge of an earlier age. While superstition and folk traditions can be seen influencing medics until surprisingly late, it is also clear that the practitioners of long ago were sometimes capable of immense sophistication. I began to collect these incredible tales from little-known corners of the medical literature: stories of weird treatments, jaw-dropping surgery and miraculous recovery from almost certain death.

The case histories in this book span three hundred years, from the early seventeenth century to the turn of the twentieth. Medicine changed dramatically during that period, undergoing a partial transformation from an art into a science. Early modern clinicians were still heavily influenced by the theories of ancient medicine, especially the writings of the Greek physician Galen—even if the realization that his opinions were not, after all, infallible had stimulated a new age of inquiry and innovation. Nevertheless, many of their treatments were based on the Galenic idea that health depends on the correct balance among four bodily fluids, or humors: blood, phlegm, yellow bile and black bile. If a surfeit of one humor was suspected, equilibrium could be restored by evacuating the excess, using bleeding or purgative medicines to do so. There was no anesthesia, so operations were short, painful and brutal—and while physicians and apothecaries had a vast range of drugs at their disposal, few were of much use.

Three centuries later, the microscope had shown that most infectious diseases were caused by organisms too small to be seen by the naked eye. Doctors had learned to control infection and perform surgery on an unconscious patient and could prescribe drugs that were effective against a range of serious conditions including heart failure and epilepsy. But old remedies still lingered: Bleeding was being recommended by some old-fashioned physicians as late as 1894, and laxatives were prescribed with wild abandon by Victorian doctors, who seldom failed to inquire about the state of their patients' bowels.

Many of the treatments offered in these stories may seem ludicrous, even barbaric, from a modern perspective, but it is worth remembering that the medics of the past were no less intelligent or assiduous than their modern counterparts. One thing that these case histories demonstrate is the admirably tenacious, even bloody-minded, determination of doctors to help their patients, in an age when their art left much to be desired. Where there were no effective remedies, they looked for new ones, and it was inevitable that many dead ends would be explored before they found the way ahead. The methods they used were consistent with their understanding of how the human body worked, and it is not their fault that medical knowledge has advanced considerably since then.

In 1851, James Young Simpson, the pioneer of chloroform anesthesia, wrote an article about the strange remedies employed by ancient Roman doctors. He cautioned that it was unwise to be too hard on the "extravagance and oddity" of their methods, adding presciently:

Perhaps, some century or two hence, our successors . . . will look back upon our present massive and clumsy doses of vegetable powders, bulky salts, nauseous decoctions, etc., with as much wonderment and surprise as we now look back upon the preceding therapeutic means of our ancestors.

The same could be said of twenty-first-century medicine, which is far from a perfected science. That said, some old treatments were misguided to the point of perversity, even by the standards of their time, and I have not resisted the urge to dole out a little gentle mockery where I thought it justified.

Most of these cases are extracted from the medical journals that started to proliferate at the end of the eighteenth century as a means for doctors to share their knowledge and experience; other source material includes surgical textbooks and newspaper reports. While a few (in the Tall Tales chapter) may be hoaxes, the vast majority are genuine case reports, written by medics who give an honest account of what they did and saw. Some are presented in their entirety; others have been edited to remove superfluous or uninteresting details; but I have not added or embellished anything.

Finally, a disclaimer: I am not a doctor, and nothing within these pages should be construed as medical advice. Readers who choose to treat their ailments by administering port-wine enemas, ingesting snake excrement or smoking cigarettes steeped in mercury do so at their own risk.

1

UNFORTUNATE PREDICAMENTS

A REGULAR FEATURE OF any hospital emergency department is the patient who turns up with an embarrassing and entirely self-inflicted complaint. When questioned about the nature of their ailment and how it came about, they may fall silent or offer a less than plausible explanation. In 1953, a man was admitted to a hospital in Barnsley with severe abdominal pain that he said had been plaguing him for almost a fortnight. Surgeons discovered severe tearing in the wall of his rectum, evidently inflicted just a few hours earlier, which they were able to repair. Asked how he had sustained this injury, the patient claimed that he was standing too near a firework "while in a stooping position," and it had gone off unexpectedly. Pressed for the truth, he admitted that he had become frustrated in his personal life and had "decided to explode a firework up his seat." That's one way of dealing with it, I suppose.

The medical literature is brimming with misguided individuals, the forebears of this proctological pyrotechnician, who inserted strange objects in places where they weren't meant to go.

One of the earliest stories concerns a monk who tried to ease his colic by coaxing a bottle of perfume inside his gut; another relates how a surgeon rescued the dignity of a farmer who had somehow ended up with a goblet wedged inside his rectum. But these are prosaic achievements compared with some of the bravura feats recorded in the following pages. What is so impressive about many of these tales of mishap is the sheer ingenuity that had gone into creating a highly regrettable situation—often matched by the imaginative manner in which a physician or surgeon went about treating the unfortunate patient.

Medicine has improved almost beyond recognition in the past few centuries, but some things never change. The human capacity for mischief, misadventure and downright idiocy is apparently a trait that progress cannot eradicate.

A FORK UP THE ANUS

Modern medical journals aren't exactly famous for their snappy headlines. The professional terminology doesn't help: It's not easy to write a zinger of a heading if the subject of your article has a name like *bestrophinopathy, idiopathic thrombocytopenic purpura* or *necrotizing fasciitis.*

But recent years have seen a fightback against such sterile jargon, with a few researchers trying to grab their readers' attention by means of literary allusions, pop culture references and bad puns. One recent article in *The New England Journal of Medicine* made a desperate pitch to George R. R. Martin fans with the headline "Game of TOR: The Target of Rapamycin Rules Four Kingdoms." Another, about foreign bodies in the bladder, was headed "From

Urethra with Shove."* And for sheer chutzpah, it's difficult to beat "Super-mesenteric-vein-expia-thrombosis, the Clinical Sequelae Can Be Quite Atrocious"—the improbable title of an article about a serious complication of appendicitis.

But my favorite medical headline of all was written almost three hundred years ago. In 1724, the *Philosophical Transactions*, the journal of the Royal Society, published a letter from Mr. Robert Payne, a surgeon from Lowestoft in Suffolk. The title is unimprovable:

III. *An Account of a Fork put up the* Anus, *that was afterwards drawn out through the Buttock; communicated in a Letter to the Publisher, by* Mr. Robert Payne, *Surgeon at* Lowestofft.

James Bishop, an apprentice to a ship-carpenter in Great Yarmouth, about nineteen years of age, had violent pains in the lower part of the abdomen for six or seven months. It did not appear to be any species of the colic; he sometimes made bloody urine, which induced Mr P. to believe it might be a stone in the bladder. He was very little relieved by physic; at length a hard tumour appeared in the left buttock, on or near the glutaeus maximus, two or three inches from the verge of the anus, a little sloping upwards. A short time after, he voided purulent matter by the anus, every day for some time.

This is the old sense of the word *tumor*: not necessarily indicating abnormal tissue growth, but a swelling of any description. This example was, as it turned out, some sort of cyst, and eventually its

---

* Groan. Urologists are notoriously awful punsters.

surface broke. The surgeon suspected it was an anal fistula—an anomalous channel between the end of the bowel and the skin. But events soon proved him wrong:

> *Shortly after the prongs of a fork appeared through the orifice of the sore, above half an inch beyond the skin. As soon as the prongs appeared, his violent pains ceased; I divided the flesh between the prongs, according to the best of my judgment; and after that made a circular incision about the prongs and so with a strong pair of pincers extracted it, not without great difficulty, handle and all entire. The end of the handle was besmeared with the excrement, when drawn out.*

Naturally. This was a surprisingly large item of cutlery:

> *It is six inches and a half long, a large pocket-fork; the handle is ivory, but is dyed of a very dark brown colour; the iron part is very black and smooth, but not rusty.*

The young man was reluctant to explain how he had managed to get himself in this predicament; at least, not until he was threatened with the withdrawal of his allowance.

> *A relation of his, a Gentleman in this neighbourhood, who sent him to be under my care, the Reverend Mr Gregory Clark, Rector of Blundeston, on whom, in a great measure, his dependence is, threatened never to look upon him more, unless he would give him an account how it came; and he told him, that, being costive,* he put the fork up his fundament, thinking by*

---

* Constipated

that means to help himself, but unfortunately it slipped up so far, that he could not recover it again.

Mr. Payne adds a postscript:

PS: He says he had no trouble or pain till a month, or more, after it was put up.

A fact that does not alter the moral of this cautionary tale: If you're constipated, it's better not to stick a fork up your fundament.

SWALLOWING KNIVES IS BAD FOR YOU

Compulsive swallowers have always featured heavily in medical literature. There are numerous cases in nineteenth-century journals—but most of the individuals concerned were obviously suffering from some kind of mental illness. This, from the *Medico-Chirurgical Transactions* for 1823, is the first I've come across in which the patient was swallowing knives for a laugh.

ACCOUNT

OF

A MAN WHO LIVED TEN YEARS,

AFTER HAVING SWALLOWED

A NUMBER OF CLASP-KNIVES;

WITH

A Description of the Appearances of the Body after Death.

By ALEX. MARCET, M.D. F.R.S. &c.

LATE PHYSICIAN TO GUY'S HOSPITAL.

In the month of June 1799, John Cummings, an American sailor, about twenty-three years of age, being with his ship on the coast of France, and having gone on shore with some of his shipmates about two miles from the town of Havre de Grace, he and his party directed their course towards a tent which they saw in a field, with a crowd of people round it. Being told that a play was acting there, they entered, and found in the tent a mountebank, who was entertaining the audience by pretending to swallow clasp-knives. Having returned on board, and one of the party having related to the ship's company the story of the knives, Cummings, after drinking freely, boasted that he could swallow knives as well as the Frenchman.

Not a particularly wise boast, and his comrades lost no time in challenging him to prove it. Eager not to disappoint them, he put his penknife in his mouth and swallowed it, washing it down with yet more booze.

The spectators, however, were not satisfied with one experiment, and asked the operator "whether he could swallow more?"; his answer was, "all the knives on board the ship", upon which three knives were immediately produced, which were swallowed in the same way as the former; and "by this bold attempt of a drunken man", (to use his own expressions) "the company was well entertained for that night."

Actions have consequences, as every sailor should know, and when foreign objects are ingested, the "consequences" usually come within twelve hours. And lo, it came to pass.*

---

* So to speak.

The next morning he had a motion, which presented nothing extraordinary; and in the afternoon he had another, with which he passed one knife, which however was not the one that he had swallowed the first. The next day he passed two knives at once, one of which was the first, which he had missed the day before. The fourth never came away, to his knowledge, and he never felt any inconvenience from it.

So no problem, right?

After this great performance, he thought no more of swallowing knives for the space of six years. In the month of March 1805, being then at Boston, in America, he was one day tempted, while drinking with a party of sailors, to boast of his former exploits, adding that he was the same man still, and ready to repeat his performance; upon which a small knife was produced, which he instantly swallowed. In the course of that evening he swallowed five more. The next morning crowds of visitors came to see him; and in the course of that day he was induced to swallow eight knives more, making in all fourteen.

It seems safe to assume at this point that Mr. Cummings was not—ahem—the sharpest knife in the drawer.

This time, however, he paid dearly for his frolic; for he was seized the next morning with constant vomiting and pain at his stomach, which made it necessary to carry him to Charleston hospital, where, as he expresses it, "betwixt that period and the 28th of the following month, he was safely delivered of his cargo."

No doubt this was a common naval euphemism of the time rather than an original *bon mot*; but it made me laugh. Having "emptied the hold," Cummings boarded a vessel traveling to France. But on the return journey, his ship was intercepted by HMS *Isis*, and he was press-ganged into service with the Royal Navy.

> *One day while at Spithead, where the ship lay some time, hav-ing got drunk and, as usual, renewed the topic of his former follies, he was once more challenged to repeat the experiment, and again complied, "disdaining," as he says, "to be worse than his word."*

An honorable person may keep their word, but a sensible one does not consume five knives, as the misguided American did that night. And he still wasn't finished; far from it.

> *On the next morning the ship's company having expressed a great desire to see him repeat the performance, he complied with his usual readiness, and "by the encouragement of the people, and the assistance of good grog", he swallowed that day, as he distinctly recollects, nine clasp-knives, some of which were very large; and he was afterwards assured by the specta-tors that he had swallowed four more, which, however, he de-clares he knew nothing about, being, no doubt, at this period of the business, too much intoxicated to have any recollection of what was passing.*

Dear oh dear. Will he never learn?

> *This, however, is the last performance we have to record; it made a total of at least thirty-five knives, swallowed at*

different times, and we shall see that it was this last attempt which ultimately put an end to his existence.

Feeling like death, and probably more than a little foolish, Cummings applied to the ship's surgeon for laxatives, but the drugs he was given had no effect.

At last, about three months afterwards, having taken a quantity of oil, he felt the knives (as he expressed it) "dropping down his bowels", after which, though he does not mention their being actually discharged, he became easier, and continued so till the 4th of June following (1806), when he vomited one side of the handle of a knife, which was recognized by one of the crew to whom it had belonged.

And who presumably was not eager to reclaim it.

In the month of November of the same year, he passed several fragments of knives, and some more in February 1807. In June of the same year, he was discharged from his ship as incurable; immediately after which, he came to London, where he became a patient of Dr Babington, in Guy's Hospital.

The doctors did not believe his story and discharged him. His health improved, and it was not until September 1808 that he reappeared:

He now became a patient of Dr Curry, under whose care he remained, gradually and miserably sinking under his sufferings, till March 1809, when he died in a state of extreme emaciation.

Even during this final illness, the doctors treating him refused to believe that he had swallowed more than thirty knives, until . . .

> *Dr Babington having one day examined him, conjointly with Sir Astley Cooper, these gentlemen concluded, from a minute inquiry into all the circumstances of the case, and especially from the deep black colour of his alvine evacuations,* that there really was an accumulation of ferruginous† matter in his organs of digestion. And this was fully confirmed soon afterwards by Mr Lucas, one of the surgeons of the hospital, who, by introducing his finger into the rectum, distinctly felt in it a portion of a knife, which appeared to lie across the intestine, but which he could not extract, on account of the intense pain which the patient expressed on his attempting to grasp it.*

The doctors tried to dissolve the knives (or at least blunt their edges) with nitric and sulfuric acids, a measure that must have done more harm than good. Powerless to help their patient, they had to watch as he wasted away and finally died. The physicians dissected his body and found that the inside of the abdomen presented an extraordinary sight: The tissues were stained a dark rusty color. Several blades were found inside the intestines, one of them piercing the colon. This alone would have been enough to kill him. But that wasn't all:

> *The stomach, viewed externally, bore evident marks of altered structure. It was not examined internally at this time, but was opened soon afterwards, in the presence of Sir Astley Cooper*

---

* Stools
† Rust-colored

and Mr Smith, surgeon of the Bristol infirmary, who happened to be present at that moment, when a great many portions of blades, knife-springs, and handles, were found in it. These fragments were between thirty and forty in number, thirteen or fourteen of them being evidently the remains of blades; some of which were remarkably corroded, and prodigiously reduced in size, while others were comparatively in a state of tolerable preservation.

A close examination of the abdominal organs also cleared up one question that had puzzled the doctors: Why was it that some knives had traveled through the gut virtually unaltered, while others had been partly digested?

When the stomach was able to expel them quickly, they passed through the intestines, enclosed within their handles, and therefore comparatively harmless; while at a later period, the knives were detained in the stomach till the handles, which were mostly of horn, had been dissolved, or at least too much reduced to afford any protection against the metallic part.

There are lessons to be learned here. Trying to impress your friends while under the influence of industrial quantities of alcohol is more often than not a really terrible idea. And more importantly, the correct answer to the question "Can you swallow more knives?" is *never* "All the knives aboard the ship."

THE GOLDEN PADLOCK

☞ *INFIBULATION, n: The action of infibulating; spec. the fastening of the sexual organs with a fibula or clasp.   [OED]*

This is not a word one encounters very often, so I had to look it up.* It seems to have made its first appearance in John Bulwer's *Anthropometamorphosis* (*Transformation of Humanity*), a treatise on tattoos, piercings and other forms of body modification published in 1650. Bulwer reveals that in ancient Greece, infibulation was used to keep young male actors chaste:

> *Among the Ancients, to prevent young effeminate inamoratos, especially comedians, from untimely venery, and cracking their voices, they were wont to fasten a ring or buckle on the foreskin of their yard.†*

I probably would have remained in blissful ignorance of this cruel practice had it not been for this entertaining article, published in *The London Medical and Physical Journal* in 1827:

> **Case of Infibulation, followed by a Schirrous Affection of the Prepuce.**
>
> *Some years ago M. Dupuytren was consulted by Dr Petroz, upon the case of M, the head of one of the most important manufactories in France.*

---

* Now that you know it, too, why not try dropping it into casual conversation?
† Penis

This is the nineteenth-century equivalent of the CEO of Airbus or Ford walking into your hospital with an embarrassing problem. And this particular "problem" was very embarrassing indeed.

> *He was about fifty years of age, of a strong and good constitution. For a long time he had had an abundant and foetid discharge from the penis: he made water with difficulty; the prepuce was much swollen, hard, and ulcerated in different parts.*

The prepuce is, of course, the foreskin. And this specimen certainly sounds as if it had seen better days.

> *So far the case presented nothing remarkable; but the curiosity of the attendants was strongly excited by observing that the prepuce had been pierced through in several places, and that the aperture and borders of these small orifices were completely covered by a perfectly-organized cutaneous tissue.*

"Perfectly-organized" means that new skin had formed over the edges of the wounds, in much the same way that an ear piercing will become lined with new skin after a few weeks, as long as an earring or stud is left inside it to keep the hole open. This observation turned out to be significant.

> *M. Dupuytren determined, before he proceeded to any decisive mode of treatment, to ascertain in what manner these perforations in the prepuce had happened. The patient stated that, when a young man, he had visited Portugal, where he had remained several years. He there formed a tender liaison with a young female of strong passions, and equally strong jealousy.*

He was devotedly attached to her, and she acquired over him the most absolute influence.

A caring relationship between a successful French businessman and his passionate Portuguese lover. How sweet.

One day during the transports of their mutual passion, he felt a slight pricking sensation in the prepuce; but, having his attention completely abstracted by the caresses of his fair mistress, he did not even examine from whence arose the disagreeable feeling he had experienced. But, on retiring from the embraces of the lady, he found the prepuce secured by a little golden padlock, beautifully made, of which she had kept the key!

Rather less sweet. It's romantic in a way, I suppose, but not the sort of gesture that everybody would appreciate.

It would appear that the lady was not deficient in eloquence, for she kept her lover in good humour by her rhetoric, assisted, indeed, by occasional caresses, and persuaded him not only to permit the padlock to remain, but to consider it a very ornamental appendage. She even gained permission to re-apply it each time, that the skin which was pierced appeared weakened; and, however incredible it may seem, she at length, "to make assurance doubly sure", put on two locks.

This seems a little excessive, and it's surprising that her paramour agreed to it. On the other hand, it may be that "M" was finding the whole thing more pleasurable than he cared to admit to his doctors.

M remained in this state for four or five years, constantly wear-
ing one or two of the locks appended to the prepuce, the key of
which was of course taken especial care of by his mistress. The
consequence ultimately was that the prepuce became diseased,
and a cancerous affection was threatened, when M. Dupuytren
was consulted.

Cancerous was sometimes used to describe persistent ulceration
rather than a malignant growth, so this may simply have been a
chronic infection in a uniquely delicate area.

The safest and most effectual course was then adopted. The pre-
puce was removed by an operation nearly resembling circumci-
sion. Under the care of M. Sanson, the cure was complete in less
than three weeks. The patient has remained in perfect health.

Let's hope that this French captain of industry managed to keep
the episode secret from his employees. It's not the sort of anecdote
you want cropping up at the staff Christmas party.

THE BOY WHO GOT HIS WICK
STUCK IN A CANDLESTICK

As the most celebrated and successful surgeon in early-nineteenth-
century France, Guillaume Dupuytren had a few things to be
proud of. He was a virtuoso technician, the master of every operation in the surgical repertoire and the inventor of several new ones.
Medical students came from all over Europe for the chance to
squeeze into the back of a lecture theater and witness his eloquence

at first hand. He became so fabulously wealthy that he once offered to lend Charles X a million francs to relieve the privations of exile.* Dupuytren was good, and he knew it. When one of his juniors complimented him on the seemingly infallible perfection of his surgery, he replied, "*Je me suis trompé, mais je crois m'être trompé moins que les autres*" ("I've made mistakes, but I think I've made fewer than everybody else").

Dupuytren's career was one studded with daring surgical feats and landmark cases. And then there's this one. Published in a Parisian journal in 1827, it appeared under a headline that translates, roughly, as "Strangulation of the Penis by a Candlestick."

Etranglement de la verge par une bobèche.

A boy, an apprentice cooper, came to the Hôtel-Dieu: from his groans, his swollen red features, his painful gait, the way he leaned while walking, stamped his feet and clutched at his genitals, one could see that he was in a great deal of pain, and that the cause of this pain was probably the urinary tract. While hastily taking off his underwear he managed to stammer that he was suffering from retention of urine, and then produced a penis which was purple, enormously swollen, and divided in the middle by a deep furrow. On separating the folds of skin which formed the edges of this depression, M. Dupuytren discovered a yellow metallic foreign body; he parted the skin further and recognised, to his amazement, the socket of a

---

* His Majesty gratefully accepted, but later wrote to Dupuytren to say that he no longer needed the cash.

candlestick, the wider end of which was facing forward, that is to say towards the pubis.

"Socket" is perhaps not the best translation for the original French word *bobèche*, which is a sort of ring or collar around the outside of a candlestick, intended to catch drips of hot wax. Or a teenage boy's penis, in this case.

The torments of the patient were terrible. He had not urinated for three days; his bladder was greatly distended and extended right up to the navel; the penis was threatened by imminent gangrene. It was essential to remove the cause of this strangulation and the retention of urine without delay. While the instruments for the operation were being prepared, the patient, who had been pressed with questions, confessed that during a debauched and drunken game he had taken the socket of his candlestick for something else, and stuck his penis in it.

Boys, eh?

Once it had been forced into the tube of this utensil he could not pull it out, and all his efforts to do so merely had the effect of increasing his misery; moreover, the sharp and narrow opening of the socket was facing forwards and pressing against the edge of the glans, which it had started to gouge.

Ouch.

M. Dupuytren first cut the wide end of the socket at two opposite points; then with considerable difficulty, because of the swelling of the parts, separated it into two portions by extending his incision. An assistant was then able to insert the smaller ends of two spatulas between the edges of the divided cylinder, which soon yielded to the efforts of the surgeon and his aide, and separated into two parts which immediately liberated the penis.

It sounds as if the operation really called for a team of firefighters rather than a surgeon. Either way, I suspect most men would demur at having cutting equipment employed in such close proximity to their, ahem, equipment. After three days without urination, the boy's bladder contents must have been at enormous pressure, so it does not take much imagination to work out what happened when that pressure was released.

M. Dupuytren learned that the strangulation had been successfully relieved when a jet of urine was projected against him.

Charming.

The patient, who was simultaneously ashamed and delighted, immediately ran off without bothering to put on his undergarments; and as he passed through the crowd he left on them—and on the square in front of Notre Dame—abundant liquid proofs of the success of the operation, which had at once removed the torments he had endured from retention of urine, as well as the danger of gangrene and even death.

As M. Dupuytren wrung out his sodden clothes, I'm sure he shared in the young man's delight.

SHOT BY A TOASTING FORK

Until the nineteenth century, most people believed that a wound to the heart meant instant death. According to centuries of tradition, the organ was the seat of the emotions, the locus of the soul and the center of the human organism. It was natural to assume that injuring this "fountain of the vital spirits" (as the sixteenth-century surgeon Ambroise Paré called it) would put an end to life. Many doctors were of the same opinion: After all, hadn't the great Galen, the most revered authority in the history of Western medicine, written that cardiac wounds were inevitably fatal? It *must* be true.

As the better class of medic knew, there was already plenty of evidence to prove otherwise. Paré himself examined the body of a duelist who had managed to run two hundred paces with a large sword wound in his heart. Others found scars in the cardiac tissue of patients who had died from natural causes—the remnants of injuries inflicted months or years earlier. Galen's assertion was thoroughly debunked, but in some quarters, it clung on stubbornly, a persistent medical myth. Cases of prolonged survival (or even recovery) after cardiac injury were still of sufficient novelty value in the 1830s to merit publication. This example, submitted to a journal in 1834 by Thomas Davis from Upton-upon-Severn in Worcestershire, is one of the best. Davis described himself as a surgeon but, like many provincial medics of the period, was in fact an apothecary without any formal qualifications.*

---

* This article prompted a furious letter from a local rival, George Sheward, alleging that Davis had plagiarized his own report of the case. Sheward waged a long campaign against Davis, which may have had its intended effect: A few years later a local business directory listed Davis not as a surgeon but as a "druggist and dealer in grain and seed"—probably a more accurate description of his occupation.

SINGULAR CASE OF A FOREIGN BODY

FOUND IN THE HEART OF A BOY.

BY THOMAS DAVIS,

Surgeon, Upton-upon-Severn.

On Saturday evening, January the 19th, 1833, I was summoned to attend William Mills, aged 10, living at Boughton, two miles from Upton. When I arrived, his parents informed me that their son had shot himself with a gun made out of the handle of a telescope toasting-fork.

Certainly an unusual way to greet a doctor. If you've decided to construct an improvised firearm, a toasting fork is unlikely to be the first implement that comes to mind.

To form the breech of the gun, he had driven a plug of wood about three inches in length into the handle of the fork. The touch hole of the gun was made after the charge of powder had been deposited in the hollow part of the handle.

Ingenious, if not particularly wise.

The consequence was that when the gunpowder exploded it forced the artificial breech, or piece of stick, from the barrel part of the gun, with such violence that it entered the thorax of the boy, on the right side, between the third and fourth ribs, and disappeared. Immediately after the accident the boy walked home, a distance of about forty yards.

The fact that he was still able to walk appeared a good sign, and when the doctor examined the boy, the case did not immediately seem a serious one.

By the time I saw him, he had lost a considerable quantity of blood, and appeared very faint; when I turned him on his right side, a stream of venous blood issued from the orifice through which the stick entered the thorax. Several hours elapsed before any degree of reaction took place. He complained of no pain.

Indeed, in the aftermath of the incident, he hardly seemed to have been affected by it.

For the first ten days or a fortnight after the accident he appeared to be recovering, and once, during that time, walked into his garden, and back, a distance of about eighty yards; and whilst there, he amused himself with his flowers, and even stirred the mould.

Hobbies: horticulture and firearms. A slightly odd combination for a ten-year-old.

He always said he was well, and was often cheerful, and even merry. There was no peculiar expression of countenance, excepting that his eyes were rather too bright. After the first fortnight he visibly emaciated, and had frequent rigors, which were always followed by faintness. The pulse was very quick. There was no cough nor spitting of blood. The secretions were healthy. He had no pain throughout his illness. He died on the

*evening of the 25th of February, exactly five weeks and two
days after the accident occurred.*

The doctor was essentially helpless to intervene. He had no way of
finding out where in the body the piece of wood had ended up, and
without anesthetics (still over a decade away), it was impossible to
perform an exploratory operation. There was an autopsy; Dr. Davis was joined by three colleagues and, strangely, the boy's father:

On opening the thorax, a small cicatrix was visible between
the cartilages of the third and fourth ribs, on the right side,
about half an inch from the sternum. The lungs appeared
quite healthy, excepting that there was a small tubercle† in the
right lung, and at its root, near to the pulmonary artery, a
small blue mark in the cellular tissue, corresponding, in size,
with the cicatrix on the parietes‡ of the chest.*

All this is consistent with a wound caused by the piece of wood,
which had apparently passed through the chest between two ribs
and entered the right lung. But then came a surprise.

*The heart, externally, appeared healthy. When an incision
was made into the heart so as to expose the right auricle and
ventricle we were astonished to find, lodged in that ventricle,
the stick which the boy had used as the breach of the gun, the one
end of it pressing against the extreme part of the ventricle, near
the apex of the heart, and forcing itself between the columnae
carneae and the internal surface of the heart; the other end*

---

* Scar
† Nodule
‡ Wall

resting upon the auriculo-ventricular valve, and tearing part
of its delicate structure, and being itself encrusted with a thick
coagulum, as large as a walnut.

The stick had lodged in the right side of the heart, the side that propels deoxygenated blood toward the lungs. The right auricle (known today as the right atrium) is the chamber by which blood enters the heart, before passing through the tricuspid (auriculo-ventricular) valve into the pumping chamber of the right ventricle. The columnae carneae (from the Latin, literally "meaty ridges") are a series of muscular columns that project into the ventricle. The stick had somehow become wedged underneath them, and a large clot had formed around it—as one would expect when a foreign body spends any length of time in the bloodstream.

We searched, in vain, for any wound, either in the heart itself,
or in the pericardium, by which the stick could have found its
way into the ventricle.

Highly significant. If the stick had simply pierced the wall of the heart, two things are likely to have happened. First, the boy would almost certainly have died within minutes: A wound big enough to admit such a large object would have caused catastrophic bleeding. Second, in the unlikely event that he had survived, it would have left a significant scar on the heart muscle.

This case strikes me as one of the most interesting on record. In
the first place, that this child should have survived such an ac-
cident as the lodgement of a stick, three inches in length, in the
right ventricle, and have been afterwards equal to so much
muscular exertion as he was, appears wonderful, especially if

we consider the mechanical difficulty which the heart had thereby to encounter in carrying on the circulation of the blood. In the next place, it appears somewhat difficult to point out how the stick found its way into the right ventricle of the heart. There was no wound, nor remnant of a wound, either in the pericardium, or in the muscular structure of the heart.

Dr. Davis now comes up with an explanation that must have seemed deeply implausible to many of his colleagues. But it's probably correct. During the First World War, surgeons encountered a number of soldiers who had a bullet in the cardiac chambers that had been swept there in the bloodstream, having entered through a blood vessel such as the vena cava (the body's largest vein, which takes deoxygenated blood back to the heart). Something similar seems to have happened in this case:

I am inclined, myself, to think that the stick, after wounding the lung, passed into the vena cava, and was carried by the stream of blood first into the right auricle, and then into the right ventricle, where it became fixed, in the manner before specified, and as is shewn in the accompanying plate.

This was indeed a remarkably interesting case, so we're lucky that the doctor took the trouble to commission an illustration. Bear in mind that the boy lived for *over a month* with this stick in situ.

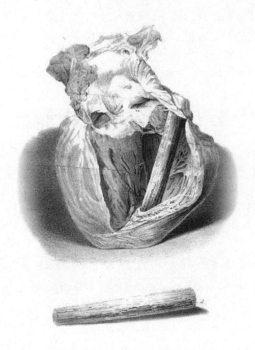

MR. DENDY'S EGGCUP CASE

Although Walter Cooper Dendy practiced as a surgeon, his most lasting contribution to the world of medicine was not an operation or instrument, but a word. In 1853, he wrote an article entitled "Psychotherapeia, or the Remedial Influence of Mind" detailing his interest in the therapeutic possibilities of the new science of psychology. Dendy's books about skin diseases and chicken pox may have been forgotten, but the discipline he named, psychotherapy, marches on.

If there's any justice in this world, he will also be remembered for a gem of a story he contributed to *The Lancet* in 1834. The heading at the top of each page refers to it simply as "Mr Dendy's Egg-Cup Case"—a splendid description of a splendid case:

> DISCOVERY OF
>
> ## A LARGE EGG-CUP
>
> IN THE
>
> ## ILEUM OF A MAN.
>
> *By* WALTER C. DENDY, *Esq.*, *M.R.C.S.L.*,
> *Stamford Street, Blackfriars.*

Mr Adams, a man 60 years of age, had been afflicted with inguinal hernia 25 years, which, although very frequently descending into the scrotum, had never been strangulated.

Even if you've no idea what this means, phrases like "descending into the scrotum" and "strangulated" make it abundantly clear that it's not much fun. An inguinal hernia is one affecting the groin. This relatively common condition occurs when part of the abdominal contents (usually a portion of intestine) drops through the inguinal canal, a passage between the abdominal cavity and the external genitalia. It usually manifests as a soft swelling around the pubic bone, although in more severe cases in men, the hernia can even protrude into the scrotum. A "strangulated" hernia is one in which the compression of local blood vessels leads eventually to tissue death.

Three months previous to his death he laboured under diarrhoea, which terminated in dysentery, from which he was partially relieved.

Dysentery, diarrhea accompanied by blood, may have been caused by some degree of strangulation. The doctors first tried using leeches, laxatives and emetics in an attempt to reduce inflammation—a regime known as the antiphlogistic plan and very much in vogue in the 1830s. If you can imagine donating blood while simultaneously throwing up and enduring constant diarrhea, you'll have a rough idea of how enjoyable it was for the patient. The initial signs in this case were encouraging; but then . . .

About a week subsequent to this the acute symptoms returned, with other signs, indicating strangulation or obstruction, such as stercoraceous vomiting and singultus, tumefaction of the abdomen, etc.—the bowels however repeatedly ejecting very scanty fluid evacuations.

Stercoraceous is an unpleasant word for an unpleasant phenomenon: The patient was vomiting what appeared to be feces. *Singultus* is an unnecessary piece of medical jargon meaning "hiccups." Mr. Dendy knew that such symptoms indicated that the small intestine was blocked, so he had another look at the hernia to see if he could identify the affected part of the gut.

On minute examination I discovered a very small knuckle of intestine deeply situated, which appeared to be intimately adherent to the mouth of the sac. As there was in this tumour extreme tenderness, I did not hesitate, after a brief endeavour to return it by the taxis, to propose an immediate operation.

Taxis is manipulation. Strangulated hernia is a medical emergency that is rarely, if ever, resolved without surgical intervention; Mr. Dendy's instincts were absolutely correct.

The friends consented, but the patient refused, stating no reason but that he did not like to be cut.

In 1833, this certainly would have been a frightening prospect, but the patient may have had other reasons for declining the operation, as it later transpired.

I therefore contented myself with palliative means, having by repeated gentle pressure returned the knuckle to the mouth of the sac, after which the stercoraceous vomiting ceased.

A positive sign, but deceptive.

He sank gradually, the abdomen becoming more and more distended, and on the 4th of December he died at three p.m., without having at any time during his illness made the slightest allusion to the circumstance which was eventually proved to have been the essential cause of his severe disorder.

This "circumstance" became clear as soon as Mr. Dendy performed a postmortem: The man's bowels contained an unexpected item of crockery.

On opening the abdomen the small intestines were seen much distended and discoloured, and on turning the superior folds aside, my finger came in contact with a hard substance which projected through the coats of the intestine. This intestine was the cross-fold of the ileum, and on further examination we were astonished to discover, through its attenuated* coats, an

---

* Thinned or wasted

earthenware eggcup closely impacted within it—the bevelled and indented edge of the cup resting on the spine—the broken stem of the cup, which projected through the bowel, near the crista of the left ilium.

The "crista," or crest, of the ilium is the curved part at the top of the pelvic bone. The eggcup had actually pierced the intestine— at this date, an inevitably fatal injury, as the gut contents would rapidly cause infection. Mr. Dendy found that there were therefore two separate injuries to the bowel: the hernia and the puncture caused by the eggcup. Naturally enough, he was keen to establish how this unusual foreign object had found its way into the patient's small intestine.

I therefore requested my friend, Mr Stephens (as I was engaged with my pencil at this point), to trace the colon from the caecum downwards.

The cecum is a blind pouch at the junction of the small and large intestines.

This inspection demonstrated the whole course of the large intestines to be in a comparatively healthy condition. The small intestines, on the contrary, the ileum especially, were extremely distended and discoloured—the graduated tints of crimson and dull purple evincing long-continued disease, which was still further confirmed by numerous patches of ulceration.

What does this tell us about the eggcup's likely route of ingress? Let's face it, the options for eggcup self-insertion are somewhat limited. Mr. Dendy concluded that the patient had swallowed the item of breakfast crockery rather than inserting it through the anus, his reasoning being that the lower part of the gut appeared healthy, while the small intestine was obviously diseased. But, as he admits, most people would be incapable of getting such a large object past the back of the throat. Mr. Dendy dismisses this objection to his theory with the observation that the circumstances "render it one of the most curious instances of which we have any record."*

I suspect that most modern experts would agree, if only on psychological grounds, that it's far more likely that a patient would stick an eggcup up their bottom than swallow it. This would also explain why the unfortunate patient was so unwilling to mention the large foreign body lodged in his gut. The article concludes with a drawing of the eggcup (presumably the work of Mr. Dendy, who was a talented artist), complete with its charmingly naïve decoration.

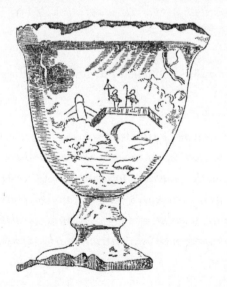

---

* In the annals of eggcup lore, certainly

It's obviously one of the imitation Chinese designs that became enormously popular toward the end of the eighteenth century: This particular example is a pattern called Broseley, which was used by many china and porcelain manufacturers of the period. But there is one quirk of the design that may permit an even more specific identification: The figures crossing the bridge are holding a parasol and a shepherd's crook. Of all the firms that used the Broseley pattern, only one seems to have included these props: Rathbone, a company active in the Staffordshire Potteries between 1812 and 1835. We may be no nearer to understanding how Mr. Dendy's patient came to have an eggcup inside his small intestine, but at least we know where it came from.

BROKEN GLASS AND BOILED CABBAGE

A significant proportion of the strangest medical cases on record fall neatly into a category we might call "unbelievably stupid things done by young men." As a student, I made my own contribution to this sizable canon when I somehow contrived to burn my nose while ironing a shirt.*

An even more idiotic self-inflicted injury was recorded in a book about emergency medicine published in 1787 by the anatomist Antoine Portal, personal physician to Louis XVIII and the founder of the French Royal Academy of Medicine. In a chapter dealing with the accidental ingestion of various dangerous substances, he recalls his inventive treatment of one particularly tricky patient:

---

* Don't ask.

SUR LES ALTÉRATIONS

Que peuvent produire dans l'Homme les chaux , les terres abforbantes & les corps vitrifiés.

I saw a young man who during a drinking bout challenged his companions to swallow a part of his glass; he broke fragments from his glass with his teeth and then swallowed them; but not with impunity.

One would rather expect there to be consequences of some kind.

He was soon seized with frightful cardialgia;* convulsive movements came on, and fears were entertained for the life of this giddy-headed young fellow, when his friends came for me.

Giddy-headed seems quite mild under the circumstances.

I first had him bled; but as the principal object of the treatment was to extract the glass which caused the symptoms, I was much embarrassed as to the means of doing so. On the one hand, I saw that tartar emetic would increase the irritation and contraction of the stomach, and that the glass would get more closely into its parietes; on the other hand, purgatives would drive the glass into the intestinal canal, the long extended surfaces of which would probably become excoriated.

---

* Heartburn

A subtle and suitably cautious train of thought. There were only two options: The glass had to be either vomited out or evacuated through the anus. Portal knew that he could use tartar emetic to provoke vomiting, but he also realized that the muscular contractions could drive the shards of glass through the stomach wall. The alternative was even worse: If the glass were allowed to get any lower into the digestive tract, with its many coils and turns, it would certainly cause a massive hemorrhage. A dilemma indeed. The solution he came up with was beautifully ingenious:

> *I thought it right, therefore, to advise the patient to fill his stomach with some food which might serve as a recipient to the glass, and then to produce vomiting. Some cabbages were procured and boiled; the patient ate a considerable quantity of them, and I then gave him two grains of tartar emetic in a glass of water.*

I'd love to know how many cabbages constituted "a considerable quantity," but I'm guessing it was more than two. Let's hope the patient liked cabbage.

> *The patient soon vomited, and threw up a considerable quantity of glass among the cabbage. He subsequently took a good deal of milk, was put into a bath, and had some emollient clysters.*

Physicians of the period had a bewildering variety of formulations for their enemas, or clysters, as they were generally known. One writer distinguishes between eight types, known as purgative, emetic, tonic, exciting, diffusible, narcotic, laxative and emollient. An "emollient" (softening) clyster was, in the words of one authority, "called for in dysentery and other diseases attended with much irritability of the bowels." There were apparently as many recipes for preparing it as there were doctors using it. The eighteenth-century physician Richard Brookes used palm oil, cow's milk and an egg yolk; Richard Reece's *Medical Guide* (1828) suggests that it should include "gelatinous and oily articles, as the decoction of the roots and leaves of the marshmallow, linseed, barley, starch, calves' feet and flesh, hartshorn shavings, etc."; Thomas Mitchell's *Materia Medica and Therapeutics* (1857), on the other hand, declares that

> *From two to four ounces of fresh butter, or the same quantity of sweet oil, in a half-pint of thin starch or slippery elm infusion, will make a good emollient clyster. An ounce of mutton suet well grated and boiled in a pint of milk will give an excellent injection, and one that has been very useful in dysenteric affections.*

None of these preparations sounds terribly pleasant. Nevertheless, for Portal's patient, it seems to have done the trick:

> *As he had become very lean in spite of these methodical aids, I advised him to drink asses' milk, which he did for more than a month, and which restored him to his former state of health.*

Cabbage and asses' milk make rather unlikely therapeutic bedfellows, but Dr. Portal clearly knew what he was doing.

HONKING LIKE A GOOSE

Humans have a remarkable capacity for misadventure, and over the years almost any object you care to think of has been extracted from some patients' airways. Nails, nuts, leeches, sheep's teeth, bullets, even part of a walking stick: All these objects and more were recorded within the space of a few years in the early nineteenth century.

But I think the following tale takes the prize for sheer outlandishness. In 1850, *The British and Foreign Medico-Chirurgical Review* printed a report by a German surgeon, Karl August Burow. A professor at the University of Königsberg, Burow was a pioneer of facial reconstruction and invented the Burow triangle, a technique still used by plastic surgeons today. Though this case report shows a certain ingenuity, it cannot claim quite the same historical significance, for the object he was asked to remove from a patient's throat was . . . another throat. A goose's throat, to be precise:

On the Removal of the Larynx of a Goose from that of a Child by Tracheotomy. By Dr. Burow.

The children in Dr Burow's vicinity are very fond of blowing through the larynx of a recently-killed goose, in order to produce some imitation of the sound emitted by this animal.

An odd pastime, but it's better than selling drugs or robbing little old ladies, I suppose.

A boy aged 12, while so engaged, was seized with a cough and swallowed the instrument; a sense of suffocation immediately

ensued, which was after a while replaced by great dyspnoea.*
Dr Burow found him labouring under this eighteen hours af-
ter, his face swollen, of a bluish-red colour, and covered with
perspiration. At every inspiration the muscles of the neck con-
tracted spasmodically, and a clear, whistling sound was heard;
and at each expiration, a hoarse sound, not very unlike that of
a goose, was emitted.

Overlooking the fact that his life was in danger, I must admit that I
would like to have heard a child honking like a goose.

As on passing the finger down to the rima glottides† it was
found closed, Dr Burow felt convinced (improbable as, from
the relative size of the two bodies, it seemed) that the larynx of
the goose had passed through it. Tracheotomy was at once per-
formed; but owing to the homogeneousness of structure of the
foreign body and of the parts it was in contact with, the great-
est difficulty existed in distinguishing it by the forceps.

Tracheotomy is one of the oldest surgical procedures known, described by many ancient authors. In this case the inhaled goose
larynx (a phrase I never expected to write) had entirely obstructed
the boy's airway, so making an incision in the throat to help him
breathe was the sensible thing to do.

Moreover, so sensitive was the mucous membrane that the in-
stant an instrument touched it, violent efforts at vomiting

---

* Difficulty in breathing
† The opening between the vocal cords

were produced, and the entire larynx was drawn up behind the root of the tongue. At last, after repeated attempts, Dr Burow having fixed the larynx in the neck by his forefinger so that it could no longer be drawn up on these occasions, he contrived to remove the entire larynx of the animal. The child was quite well by the ninth day.

Tracheotomies were fraught with danger in this era, since postoperative infections were common. This was undoubtedly an excellent result.

Dr Burow says that it was a matter of great congratulation for him that many pupils were present during this operation, and thus able to confirm the correctness of a statement so incredible as to stand much in need of such confirmation.

Well, it's certainly an unlikely thing to happen; but, on the other hand, who'd make up something like that?

PENIS IN A BOTTLE

Most doctors have found themselves treating a patient with injuries so embarrassing that they are unwilling or unable to provide a plausible explanation. In his book *Urological Oddities* (1948), the American physician Wirt Bradley Dakin gives a number of feeble excuses provided by patients with strange objects stuck in their bladders, ranging from "I was taking my temperature and it slipped from my grasp" (a thermometer) to "I wanted to see what would happen" (a six-foot coil of wire). Others declined to proffer any explanation, such as the "dignified and prominent citizen" who sought treatment after introducing an earthworm into his own urethra.*

Just occasionally, however, an outlandish-sounding excuse turns out to be entirely truthful. Just such a case was reported in 1849 by Dr. Azariah Shipman, a surgeon from Syracuse in New York. When summoned to treat a young man with a glass bottle stuck on his penis, he was probably not expecting the scenario to have a perfectly innocent explanation:

NOVEL EFFECTS OF POTASSIUM—FOREIGN BODIES IN THE URE-THRA—CATALEPSY.

A few months ago I was called in great haste to a young gentleman, who was in a most ludicrous yet painful condition. I found on examination a bottle holding about a pint, with a short neck and small mouth, firmly attached to his body by the penis, which was drawn through the neck and projected into the bottle, being swollen and purple. The bottle, which was a white one, with a ground-glass stopper and perfectly transparent, had an opening of three fourths of an inch in diameter only; and the penis being much swollen rendered its extraction utterly impossible. The patient was greatly frightened, and so urgent for its removal that he would give me no account of its getting into its present novel situation, but implored me to liberate it instantly, as the pain was intense and the mental anguish and fright intolerable.

---

* To be fair, if there was ever an appropriate moment to plead the fifth, this was probably it.

I think if I sought medical assistance in such a condition, I would also be hoping for treatment first, explanation second.

> *Seeing no hopes of getting an explanation in his present predicament, and after endeavouring to pull the penis out with my fingers without success, I seized a large knife lying on the table, and with the back of it I struck a blow on the neck of the bottle, shivering it to atoms and liberating the penis in an instant, much to the delight of the terrified youth.*

The tip of the newly liberated member was enormously swollen and black, and blistered as if it had been burned in a fire. As for its owner:

> *He complained of smarting and pain in the penis, after the bottle was removed; and inflammation, swelling and discoloration continued for a number of days, but by scarification* and cold applications, subsided; yet not without great apprehensions on the part of the patient, and a good degree of real pain in the penis. The reader is probably anxious to know, by this time, how a penis, belonging to a live man, found its way into so unusual a place as the mouth of a bottle.*

I have no doubt that everybody who has ever read this case report in the 165 years since it was written has wondered exactly this.

> *I was extremely curious myself; but the fright and perturbation of the patient's mind, and his apprehensions of losing his penis entirely, either by the burn, swelling, inflammation, or*

---

* A mild form of bloodletting by means of superficial scratches

by my cutting it off to get it out of the bottle, all came upon him at once and overwhelmed him with fear.

That's one possible reason for his reticence, certainly.

Now for the explanation. A bottle in which some potassium had been kept in naphtha,* and which had been used up in experiments, was standing in his room; and wishing to urinate without leaving his room, he pulled out the glass stopper and applied his penis to its mouth. The first jet of urine was followed by an explosive sound and flash of fire, and quick as thought the penis was drawn into the bottle with a force and tenacity which held it as firmly as if in a vice. The burning of the potassium created a vacuum instantaneously, and the soft yielding tissue of the penis effectually excluding the air, the bottle acted like a huge cupping glass to this novel portion of the system. The small size of the mouth of the bottle compressed the veins, while the arteries continued to pour their blood into the glans, prepuce, etc. From this cause, and the rarefied air in the bottle, the parts swelled and puffed up to an enormous size.

A very serious situation. And *not at all* funny.

How much potassium was in the bottle at the time is not known, but it is probable that but a few grains were left, and those broken off from some of the larger globules, and so small as to have escaped the man's observation. I was anxious to test the matter (though not with the same instruments which the patient had done) . . .

---

* A flammable liquid hydrocarbon

I'm glad to hear that, at least.

> *. . . and for that purpose took a few small particles of potassium, mixed with about a teaspoonful of naphtha, and placed them in a pint bottle. Then I introduced some urine with a dash, while the end of one of my fingers was inserted into the mouth of the bottle, but not so tightly as to completely close it, and the result was a loud explosion like a percussion cap, and the finger was drawn forcibly into the bottle and held there strongly—thus verifying, in some degree, this highly interesting philosophical experiment, which so frightened my friend and patient.*

This sounds entirely plausible. In case you haven't seen what happens when a stream of urine hits a piece of potassium, it is every bit as dramatic as Dr. Shipman describes. The metal is highly reactive and even a small fragment will explode violently when thrown into water. It also oxidizes rapidly in air, which is why the young chemistry enthusiast kept his samples under naphtha.

> *The novelty of this accident is my apology for spending so many words in reporting it, while its ludicrous character will, perhaps, excite a smile; but it was anything but a joke at the time to the poor sufferer, who imagined in his fright that if his penis was not already ruined, breaking the bottle to liberate it would endanger its integrity by the broken spicules* cutting or lacerating the parts.*

---

* Sharp splinters

Once you've dried your tears of mirth, perhaps you'll spare a thought for the poor fellow.

THE COLONIC CARPENTRY KIT

In 1840 an Irish visitor to Brest in northern France was given a tour of the local prison. It was a vast edifice built to accommodate six thousand inmates and, at its peak, contained a tenth of the city's population. The prisoners were also slaves: Condemned to hard labor, they provided a large and reluctant workforce whose employment ranged from large-scale construction work to making sails. Opened in 1751, the building was innovative in its design, constructed in such a way that even in their cells the inmates were under constant surveillance from their guards. Nevertheless, as Andrew Valentine Kirwan observed, the prison was still a hotbed of

> *every crime and every vice, where the indifferent become bad,*
> *and the bad, unabashed and unamended, become daily worse.*

Kirwan quickly learned that, far from being a place of moral correction, the jail had become a sort of finishing school for those wishing to perfect their education in the criminal arts. But instead of deportment and flower arranging, the crooks were taking classes in housebreaking and deception:

> *The forger learns from the thief the art of making a false key,*
> *and the thief in return is initiated into the mystery of counter-*
> *feiting signatures.*

This was not a pleasant place to live: The work was hard, the diet poor and the death toll appallingly high. Unsurprisingly, prisoners made frequent attempts to escape. Kirwan witnessed a thriving trade in replica keys, counterfeit passports and other paraphernalia needed by the would-be fugitive. Few, however, went to the lengths of the convict who became the unwitting subject of an article in the *Medical Times*:*

FOREIGN BODY IN THE COLON TRANSVERSUM.

A very curious case of this affection occurred a short time ago in the bagno of Brest.

The term *bagno* (usually *bagne* in French) was used in southern European countries to describe a prison whose inmates were made to perform hard labor.

A dangerous convict, who had already once escaped from prison, suddenly complained of abdominal pain, constipation, sickness, fever, etc. No hernia could be found, but the symptoms, which soon increased in severity, left no doubt of the existence of an internal incarceration of the bowel.

The doctor suspected that a loop of intestine had become trapped. This was potentially very serious: If its blood supply had been cut off, the tissue would quickly die, resulting in gangrene.

---

* Strangely, this article appeared three years after the prison had been permanently closed and its inmates transported to a penal colony in Guyana.

The vomiting became obstinate, the pain very intense, and the meteorism considerable.

Meteorism (also known as tympanites) is a condition in which the abdomen becomes tight and distended. It is caused by a buildup of gas in the intestinal tract—a classic symptom of bowel necrosis.

As the patient, in spite of treatment, continued to grow worse, he confided at last to his medical attendant that he had placed a little leathern bag with money in the rectum, in order to hide it from the gaoler. An examination of the rectum was then made, but nothing was found in it.

The prisoner was not, it transpired, being entirely truthful. Having tried to conceal the self-inflicted nature of his malady, he now resorted to another lie. Yes, he had stuck something up his bottom—but not a purse.

The symptoms continually increased, and after a time a tumour became visible at the left side of the abdomen, corresponding to the site of the descending colon. The convict, at this stage of the disease, said that he had introduced an étui of wood into the rectum, and having been surprised, he had, in the hurry, placed it with the top upwards, instead of with the bottom.

The truth, at last! An *étui* is a small ornamental case used to carry personal effects such as penknives or a sewing kit; many surgeons used them to carry their instruments. This example was not symmetrical, since one end was apparently easier to get a grip on than the other. Why the patient thought it less embarrassing to have inserted a purse up his own bottom than a wooden case remains a mystery.

A week after the onset of symptoms, the prisoner died, and a postmortem was carried out. The surgeon who performed it found that the patient had suffered acute peritonitis; the bowel was "immensely distended by gas." But the strangest finding was in the colon, where

> *a voluminous foreign body was found, which proved to be a cylindrico-conical box, the conical end of which looked towards the caecum.* The box consisted of two pieces of sheet-iron, was about 6 inches long and 5 inches broad, weighed nearly 22 ounces, and was covered by a piece of skin, no doubt for protecting the mucous membrane of the rectum from the contact with the metal, and for facilitating the expulsion of the box.*

This was a seriously large object to be lodged in anybody's intestine. When the medics opened the box, they found it contained the following:

> *A piece of a gun-barrel, four inches long.*
> *A screw of steel.*
> *A mother-screw also of steel.*
> *A screw-driver; from which four instruments a pulley may be formed strong enough for removing iron railings.*
> *A saw of steel for cutting wood, four inches long.*
> *Another saw for cutting metal.*
> *A boring syringe.*
> *A prismatic file.*

---

* I.e., toward the upper part of the bowel

One two-franc piece and four one-franc pieces tied together with thread.

A piece of tallow for oiling the instruments.

A complete escape kit, in other words. You have to admire his attention to detail, even if the execution left something to be desired.

After this extraordinary discovery had been made, an inquiry was instituted into the habits of the galley-slaves, and the chief gaoler said that convicts of the worst description used to conceal suspicious objects, as instruments, money, etc., in the rectum.

Some things never change.

These items, however, were generally of small size, being scarcely ever larger than an inch or so, and they were called 'necessaries' by the convicts.

Today's "necessaries" include the smallest cell phone on the market, an item familiar to any prison officer who has ever had to conduct an internal cavity search.

The gaoler had never seen one similar to the box just described.

I should think not!

These étuis have almost always the same shape, one extremity being conical and the other blunt. They are always introduced in such manner that the conical end looks towards the anus, whereby the expulsion of it is facilitated. In the present instance the convict had been obliged to conceal his necessaire in a hurry on the approach of a person, and confounded the ends of the étui.

Instead of sitting just inside the rectum, where it could be easily removed when nobody was looking, the box had escaped from the prisoner's grasp and made its way a surprising distance into the large intestine.

My advice? If you're planning to break out of prison, just get a friend to bake a file inside a cake.

SUFFOCATED BY A FISH

Surgeons in Pondicherry, southern India, were just about to begin a routine operation in 2004 when an urgent beeping indicated that all was not well with their patient. A fit and healthy young man, he had been under general anesthesia for only a few minutes when his heart rate plummeted and monitors showed that he was being starved of oxygen. Suspecting that the tube inserted into the patient's airways had been dislodged, the anesthetist pulled it out and started to ventilate him by hand. The man's condition quickly stabilized, but when the anesthetist looked at what he had just removed from the patient's airways, he nearly passed out in shock: Coiled around the end of the tube was the cause of the trouble—a huge parasitic worm.*

Foreign objects lodged in the airway are a common cause of hospital admission, particularly among children—but generally

---

* This story is already bad enough, but even worse is how it got there: It had migrated from the man's stomach, up his esophagus and then down the trachea toward his lungs.

speaking, the items that get into the "wrong tube" are not alive at the time. However, there are well-documented cases of worms, leeches and even fish being inhaled by mischance or misadventure— as in this "news in brief" item published in 1863:

EXTRAORDINARY DEATH.

A warder of the Bagne at Toulon has just met his death in the following manner: he was amusing himself, while off duty, with fishing in the dock, when having caught a fish about seven inches long and two broad, and not knowing where to place it while baiting his hook conceived the idea of holding it be- tween his teeth. The fish struggling in the convulsions of death, ended by slipping its head first into the mouth, and thence, ow- ing to the viscous matter with which the scales were covered, down his throat, completely filling up the cavity. The man rushed about for aid, but soon dropped dead from suffocation.

Extraordinary, but not unique. Four years earlier, a similar case had been reported in a colonial medical journal, *The Indian Lancet*:

In 1859, Dr White reported the case of a strong Madras Bheestee,* into whose mouth a fish had jumped while he was bathing. On opening the mouth, the tail of a large catfish pre- sented itself with the body firmly fixed within the fauces, and filling up the isthmus completely.

---

* In colonial India, a bheestie was a domestic servant whose job was to keep the house- hold supplied with water.

The fauces is the arch of tissue at the back of the mouth; the isthmus of the fauces is the opening it surrounds. All things considered, it's surprising he hadn't already suffocated.

It had entered flat, so that the fin of one side was posterior to the velum,* and opened out on any attempt being made to withdraw the fish. The operation of oesophagotomy was commenced and abandoned. A piece of cane was made into a probang,† and with it attempts were made to press the fish downwards into the oesophagus. It did pass downwards, when the patient at once ceased to breathe, gave one convulsive struggle, and died to all appearance.

Not so good. As soon became clear, the fish had not been pushed into the stomach as intended, but instead had become lodged in the trachea, obstructing the airway. The doctor quickly realized that the only option was to attempt a tracheotomy.

The trachea was immediately opened, and respiration was restored. In the course of the night the man coughed up the fish, the fins having become softened by decomposition.

Nice. Nevertheless, better to cough up a decomposing fish than to die because it's stuck in your throat.

Dr White states that "this is by no means an uncommon accident in India. Natives bathing and swimming, which they always do with their mouths wide open . . .

---

* Soft palate
† A long instrument, generally made from a piece of sponge on a stick, used to dislodge foreign objects in the esophagus

Really?

> "... in tanks that abound in fish, are not unfrequently brought to hospital dying from suffocation and alarm with a large catfish firmly impacted in the fauces. It is a coarse kind of fish, with long bony fins very sharp indeed at their extremities."

It seems difficult to believe that there really was an epidemic of fish inhalation in nineteenth-century India, but at least two virtually identical cases were reported over the next few years. One patient survived for an astonishing thirty-four hours with the rotting corpse of the unfortunate creature lodged in his airway. And it still happens today: A recent review found no fewer than seventy-five documented cases of live fish in the airways. After surveying the available evidence, the authors of the article make this helpful observation:

> Live fish aspiration is frequently accidental or the result of poor judgment involving placing a live fish in the mouth.

A conclusion that I suspect most readers will have reached for themselves.

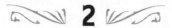

2

MYSTERIOUS ILLNESSES

HAVE YOU EVER wondered how many human diseases there are? I don't mean just the infectious ones like influenza, leprosy and bubonic plague, but also noncommunicable diseases such as diabetes and cancer and the many genetic disorders. The question is impossible to answer, since new ones are being identified all the time. The World Health Organization oversees the publication of the *International Classification of Diseases*, a terrifying compendium of pretty much everything that can go wrong with you. When the first edition of this document appeared in 1893, it identified 161 separate disorders; the tenth, published a century later, listed more than 12,000. By some estimates, doctors now recognize as many as 30,000 distinct diseases, although nobody can agree on even an approximate figure.

Some, such as HIV/AIDS or Ebola, simply did not exist a hundred years ago and emerged as a result of the evolution of new and particularly unpleasant pathogens. Others are being identified only because recent advances in gene sequencing make it possible to locate the precise mutation that causes an otherwise mystifying set of symptoms. Thousands of these conditions are classified as rare diseases, meaning that they affect less than 0.05 percent of the population—and are encountered so infrequently that treatment options are few, and often virtually untested.

Diagnosing a rare condition can pose a challenge to the most talented and experienced clinician, even one with the resources of a modern hospital at their disposal. So it is easy to sympathize with the eighteenth-century physician who visited a family in Suffolk and found them suffering from a strange and terrible disease that made their limbs wither and fall off. The illness was new to England, its cause was unknown and treatment impossible. He could do little more but try to relieve their pain and then set down the symptoms on paper so that his colleagues might recognize them in the future. I find these first encounters between a medic and a never-before-encountered adversary fascinating: You can often sense the doctor's frustration as they try to work out what they're up against.

But such descriptions of novel diseases were sometimes written for reasons less nobly scientific. In the seventeenth century, when the *Philosophical Transactions* and other early journals were founded, natural philosophers took a particular interest in monsters, deviations from the otherwise perfect productions of Nature. One typical article of this period was entitled "A Relation of Two Monstrous Pigs with the Resemblance of Human Faces, and Two Young Turkeys Joined by the Breast." The desire to understand and study such anomalies was genuine, but these accounts also played to a very human fascination with the grotesque and freakish.

While the study of "prodigies and monsters" fell out of fashion in the eighteenth century, the sensationalist instincts of journal editors persisted for long afterward. A mysterious new disease with exotic symptoms (the weirder the better) almost guaranteed publicity, even if the supporting evidence was shaky. A description of a boy who apparently vomited a fetus was of little clinical value, but it made a terrific story. Most of the strange conditions documented in this chapter were probably genuine, although even the most open-minded expert might demur at the idea that it is possible for a patient to urinate through their ear.

A HIDEOUS THING HAPPENED IN HIGH HOLBORN

Little is known about the seventeenth-century physician Edward May, except that he moved in rather elevated social circles. He came from a distinguished Sussex family that produced numerous MPs, a dean of St. Paul's Cathedral and several members of the royal household. Edward was himself apparently a regular at the court of Charles I, holding the position of physician-extraordinary to Queen Henrietta Maria. He also taught at the Musæum Minervæ, a sort of finishing school for young noblemen, whose eccentric curriculum ranged from astronomy to riding and fencing.

But the most notable episode of Dr. May's life was an incident so notorious and ghastly that one contemporary, the celebrated Welsh historian James Howell, described it as "a hideous thing that happened in High Holborn." Dr. May recorded this unsettling experience in a pamphlet published in 1639 under this rather wonderful title:

A

MOST CERTAINE

AND TRVE

RELATION

OF A STRANGE MON-

STER OR SERPENT

Found in the left Ventricle of

the heart of IOHN PENNANT, Gentle-

man, of the age of 11. yeares.

The unfortunate young patient, John Pennant (deceased), was the scion of an aristocratic Welsh family that could trace its lineage back to the Norman Conquest. Edward May sets the scene:

> *The seventh of October this year current, 1637, the Lady Her-*
> *ris wife unto Sir Francis Herris Knight, came unto me and*
> *desired that I would bring a surgeon with me, to dissect the*
> *body of her nephew John Pennant, the night before deceased, to*
> *satisfy his friends concerning the causes of his long sickness*
> *and of his death; and that his mother, to whom myself had*
> *given help some years before concerning the stone, might be as-*
> *certained whether her son died of the stone or no?*

Dr. May had previously treated the young man's mother for bladder stones, which were far more prevalent in the seventeenth century than they are today. She naturally wondered whether this was the cause of his death.

> *Upon which entreaty I sent for Master Jacob Heydon, surgeon,*
> *dwelling against the Castle Tavern behind St Clements church*

in the Strand, who with his manservant came unto me. And in a word we went to the house and chamber where the dead man lay. We dissected the natural region and found the bladder of the young man full of purulent and ulcerous matter, the upper parts of it broken, and all of it rotten; the right kidney quite consumed, the left tumefied* as big as any two kidneys, and full of sanious matter. All the inward and carnouse† parts eaten away and nothing remaining but exterior skins.

Sanious matter means bloody pus. So far, so bad; it sounds as if a catastrophic infection had wrecked his urinary system.

Nowhere did we find in his body either stone or gravel. We ascending to the vital region‡ found the lungs reasonable good, the heart more globose§ and dilated, than long; the right ventricle of an ashen colour shrivelled, and wrinkled like a leather purse without money, and not anything at all in it: the pericardium, and nervous membrane, which containeth that illustrious liquor of the lungs, in which the heart doth bathe itself, was quite dried also.

I like Dr. May's turn of phrase: "wrinkled like a leather purse" is a vivid description of a diseased heart. The "illustrious liquor of the lungs" is pericardial fluid, whose main function is to lubricate the outer surface of the heart as it beats. In a healthy patient the pericardium, the tough sac surrounding the heart, normally contains a few teaspoons (around 50 milliliters) of this fluid.

---

* Swollen
† Fleshy
‡ I.e., the thorax
§ Round

The left ventricle of the heart, being felt by the surgeon's hand,
appeared to him to be as hard as a stone, and much greater
than the right; wherefore I wished Mr Heydon to make inci-
sion, upon which issued out a very great quantity of blood; and
to speak the whole verity, all the blood that was in his body left,
was gathered to the left ventricle, and contained in it.

A common observation in early autopsy reports was that the major
vessels were empty, leading some authorities to suggest that the
blood somehow "retreated" to the heart after death. In reality, in
the absence of a heartbeat, the blood obeys gravity, sinking to the
lowest point of the body. In forensic pathology, this can offer a useful indication as to whether a body has been moved after death.
Back to Dr. May:

No sooner was that ventricle emptied, but Mr Heydon still com-
plaining of the greatness and hardness of the same, myself
seeming to neglect his words, because the left ventricle is thrice
as thick of flesh as the right is in sound men for conservation of
vital spirits, I directed him to another disquisition: but he
keeping his hand still upon the heart, would not leave it, but
said again that it was of a strange greatness and hardness.

Dr. May correctly points out that in a healthy human heart the
muscle of the left ventricle, or pumping chamber, is approximately
three times thicker than that of the right. This is because it oper-
ates at higher pressure, pumping oxygenated blood to the whole
body, whereas the right ventricle must propel deoxygenated blood
only as far as the lungs. But in this case the left ventricle was even
larger than normal. This was almost certainly left ventricular hy-
pertrophy, a thickening of the heart muscle. It has several possible

causes, and its presence suggests that the man had been ill for some time, since it takes a while to develop.

Dr. May asked the surgeon to make a larger incision in the ventricle:

> . . . *by which means we presently perceived a carnouse substance, as it seemed to us wreathed together in folds like a worm or serpent; at which we both much wondered, and I entreated him to separate it from the heart, which he did, and we carried it from the body to the window, and there laid it out.*

When May examined this object in daylight, he had quite a shock.

> *The body was white, of the very colour of the whitest skin of man's body: but the skin was bright and shining, as if it had been varnished over; the head all bloody, and so like the head of a serpent, that the Lady Herris then shivered to see it, and since hath often spoken it, that she was inwardly troubled at it, because the head of it was so truly like the head of a snake. The thighs and branches were of flesh colour, as were also all these fibres, strings, nerves, or whatsoever else they were.*

I wasn't aware that snakes had thighs. Dr. May was at first skeptical that a human heart could contain a snake, and wondered aloud whether it might just be a "pituitose and bloody collection"—in other words, a large mass of blood and phlegm. This conjecture we will return to later. He decided to examine the strange creature more closely.

> *I first searched the head and found it of a thick substance, bloody and glandulous about the neck, somewhat broken (as I*

conceived) by a sudden or violent separation of it from the
heart, which yet seemed to me to come from it easily enough.
The body I searched likewise with a bodkin between the legs or
thighs, and I found it perforate, or hollow, and a solid body,
to the very length of a silver bodkin, as is here described; at
which the spectators wondered.

Following the surgeon's lead, the bystanders took it in turns to
probe the "snake" with a metal bodkin, until they were all convinced that the object before them was a worm, serpent or other
creature, with identifiable anatomical features including a digestive tract. Evidently aware that they might not be believed, they
signed an affidavit confirming what they had seen.

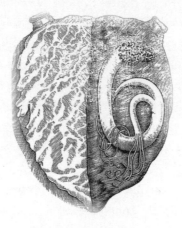

Snake inside the heart of John Pennant, from Edward May's
A most certaine and true Relation *(1639)*

Was there really a snake inside the young man's heart, or perhaps a
worm? Almost certainly not. You may recall that Dr. May's first
thought was that the strange object was a "bloody collection"; in
other words, a large clot. This seems far more likely, and two

centuries later, a notable Victorian physician came to the same conclusion.

Benjamin Ward Richardson was a diligent and original researcher who discovered several novel anesthetic agents as well as
the first effective drug for the treatment of angina pain, amyl nitrite.
He also had a particular interest in the formation of thrombi, or
blood clots. In December 1859, he gave a series of lectures* about
the formation of "fibrinous depositions"—clots—inside the heart.
Richardson noted that thrombi come in all shapes and sizes: Sometimes they form long filaments or even hollow tubes, with blood
continuing to flow through a central channel. He suggested that
this is precisely what Dr. May had found inside the young man's
heart: a monster clot that had grown to look like some sort of myth-
ical serpent.

Assuming it was a clot, we can now make a tentative guess at a
diagnosis. You'll recall that the original surgeon remarked upon
the unusual "greatness and hardness" of the left ventricle of the
heart. Not only was the muscle hypertrophied (increased in size),
but it had become unnaturally rigid. This is something often seen
in the case of a rare blood disorder, hypereosinophilic syndrome
(HES), which is also associated with a high risk of extensive clot-
ting in the heart. HES can also attack multiple organs simultaneously, which would explain the state of the young man's kidneys.
It's impossible to be sure, of course, but the symptoms certainly
seem to fit.

You may be wondering what happened to the "serpent" after
the postmortem had been completed. Dr. May explains that the

---

* His unfortunate students were required to give up their Christmas vacations in order to
attend them. "I know that it may be considered, by indolent men, as no charitable act on
my part to break in upon your holiday time," said Richardson. "At the same time, I offer
no apology for the act." Merry Christmas, guys!

surgeon was keen to hold on to it for further study, but the dead man's mother had other ideas:

> *The surgeon had a great desire to conserve it, had not the mother desired that it should be buried where it was born, saying and repeating, "As it came with him, so it shall go with him"; wherefore the mother staying in the place, departed not, till she had seen him sew it up again into the body after my going away.*

As Nietzsche's protagonist puts it in *Also sprach Zarathustra*: "You have evolved from worm to man, but much within you is still worm."

THE INCREDIBLE SLEEPING WOMAN

Sometime in the 1750s (the precise date is unknown), a group of London doctors decided to get together periodically to discuss their own cases and any novel developments in medical practice. The enterprise was inspired by the foundation in 1731 of the Edinburgh Medical Society, though the London group never acquired a formal name.* It produced an occasional journal, the *Medical Observations and Inquiries*, intended to disseminate the society's research to a wider audience. Its purpose was thoroughly modern: to improve medicine through evidence-based research, as the preface to the first volume, published in 1757, explained:

> *The persons who formed this Society were either such as had the care of hospitals, or were otherwise in some degree of repute*

---

* They identified themselves simply as "a society of physicians in London."

in their profession; and consequently had frequent opportuni-
ties of making observations themselves, and of verifying, in the
course of their practice, the discoveries of others.

One of the cases included in the first installment of the *Medical
Observations and Inquiries* was this strange tale:

> **XXII.** *An Account of an extraordinary sleepy
> Woman, near* Mons *in* Hainault. *By
> Dr.* Terence Brady, *Physician to His
> Royal Highness Prince* Charles *of* Lorraine.
> *Read May* 3, 1756.

*Elizabeth Orvin, born at St Gilain, of a healthy robust consti-
tution, served the curate of that place for many years very
faithfully, till the beginning of 1738, that she became very sul-
len, uneasy, and so surly, that the neighbours said she was losing her senses. Towards the month of August, she fell into an
extraordinary sleep, which lasted four days; during which
time, she took no manner of nourishment, neither was it possible to rouse her.*

Mme. Orvin did eventually wake up, but for the next ten years, she
routinely slept for seventeen hours a day, from 3 A.M. till 8 P.M., and
was usually awake only at night. Dr. Brady visited her in February
1756, and found her fast asleep at five o'clock in the afternoon. She
was as stiff as a board and could not be roused:

> *I put my mouth to her ear, and called as loud as I could, but
> could not wake her; and to be sure that there was no cheat in the
> matter, I thrust a pin through her skin and flesh to the bone.*

Well, that escalated quickly.

I kept the flame of burning paper to her cheek till I burned the scarff skin,* and put volatile spirits and salts into her nose, and lastly, thrust a little linen dipped in rectified spirit of wine in her nostril, and kindled it for a moment: all this was done without my being able to observe the least change in her countenance, or signs of feeling.

Methods not—as far as I know—currently used by any reputable sleep clinic. Three hours later the woman awoke:

About eight, she turned in her bed, got up abruptly, and came to the fire. I asked her several questions, to which she gave surly answers. She was gloomy and sad, and repeated often, that she would rather be out of the world, than in such a state. I could get no satisfactory account from her, about her sickness; all that I could learn from her was, that she felt a heaviness in her head, which she knew to be the forerunner of her disorder, and which determined her to go to bed, where she lay without once turning, from the time she lay down till her sleep was over, and had, during that time, no sort of evacuation except by perspiration.

On occasions she slept for so long that she had to be fed (while still asleep) through a funnel. The local doctor told Dr. Brady about some of the enterprising, but barbaric, methods they had adopted in attempts to wake her up. These entailed her . . .

---

* An archaic term for the outermost layer of skin. To "burn the scarff skin" implies the formation of a blister.

... being whipped till the blood ran down her shoulders, of her having her back rubbed with honey, and her being exposed in a hot day before a hive of bees, where she was stung to such a degree that her back and shoulders were full of little lumps or tumours. At other times, they thrust pins under her nails, together with some other odd experiments that I must pass over in silence, on account of their indecency.

The mind boggles. Even the mildest of these techniques arguably crosses the line separating therapy from abuse. Nevertheless, she remained, to all appearances, beyond the help of medicine.

This poor woman is now fifty-five years of age, of a pale colour, and not very lean. She never sees daylight, but sleeps out the longest day in summer; and, in winter, begins to sleep several hours before day, and does not awake till two or three hours after sunset.

This seems to have been an isolated case; but what's interesting about the report is that the woman's symptoms very much resemble those of Encephalitis lethargica, a mysterious illness that began to sweep across much of the globe at around the time of the First World War. Patients often fell into a deep sleep from which they could not be roused. When epidemiologists looked back through historical records, they found that several similar outbreaks had occurred in earlier centuries. Unexplained bouts of somnolence plagued the residents of Copenhagen in 1657, London in 1673, Germany in 1712 and France in 1776. What caused the illness is unknown, although it often seemed to accompany epidemics of influenza. We'll never know what was wrong with the Sleepy Woman of Mons. But it's just possible that she had an unusual variety of flu.

THE DREADFUL MORTIFICATION

A case published in the *Philosophical Transactions* in 1762 is a reminder of a world we have thankfully left behind: one in which disease could rapidly maim or kill entire families, while doctors looked on helplessly. Life was often, in the philosopher Thomas Hobbes's phrase, "solitary, poor, nasty, brutish and short." Hobbes was writing about war, but disease was as formidable an enemy as the eighteenth century could muster.

This report was written by Charlton Wollaston, a twenty-nine-year-old who had just been appointed physician to the queen's household. His promising career was cut tragically short two years later when he died from a fever. His daughter Mary later attributed his death to blood poisoning contracted when "opening a mummy, he having previously by accident cut a finger."

> LXXXIII. *Extract of a Letter from* Charlton Wollaston, *M. D. F. R S. to* William Heberden, *M. D. F R. S. dated* Bury St. Edmund's, April 1 3, 1762, *relating to the Case of Mortification of Limbs in a Family at* Wattisham *in* Suffolk.

John Downing, a poor labouring man who lives at Wattisham, a small village about sixteen miles from Bury, in January last had a wife and six children; the eldest a girl of fifteen years of age, the youngest about four months. They were also at that time very healthy, as the man himself, and his neighbours, assured me. On Sunday 10th January, the eldest girl complained in the morning of a pain in her left leg; particularly in the calf of the leg. Towards evening the pain grew exceedingly violent.

The same evening another girl, about ten years old, complained of the same violent pain in the leg. On the Monday the mother and another child, and on the Tuesday all the rest of the family, except the father, were affected in the same manner. The pain was exceedingly violent; insomuch, that the whole neighbour-hood was alarmed with the loudness of their shrieks.

Chilling. This was a rapid, insidious and deeply unpleasant complaint. Dr. Wollaston visited the family and questioned them in detail about the progress of the disease.

In about four, five, or six days, the diseased leg began to grow less painful, and to turn black gradually; appearing at first covered with spots, as if it had been bruised. The other leg began to be affected, at that time, with the same excruciating pain, and in a few days that also began to mortify.

To "mortify" means to become gangrenous: The leg discolored and then went black as the tissue died.

The mortified parts separated, without assistance, from the sound parts, and the surgeon had in most of the cases no other trouble than to cut through the bone, with little or no pain to the patient.

The summary that follows is simply written, but brutal in its impact.

Mary, the mother, aged forty. The right foot off at the ankle; the left leg mortified, a mere bone; but not off.

Mary, aged fifteen. One leg off below the knee: the other perfectly sphacelated,* but not yet off.
Elizabeth, aged thirteen, both legs off below the knees.
Sarah, aged ten, one foot off at the ankle.
Robert, aged eight, both legs off below the knees.
Edward, aged four, both feet off at the ankles.
An infant four months old, dead.

Only the father escaped relatively unscathed: A couple of fingers became stiff and useless, but his lower extremities were not affected.

It is remarkable, that during all the time of this calamity, the whole family are said to have appeared in other respects well. They ate heartily, and slept well when the pain began to abate. When I saw them, they all seemed free from fever, except the girl, who has an abscess in her thigh. The mother looks emaciated, and has very little use of her hands. The rest of the family seemed well. One poor boy, in particular, looked as healthy and florid as possible, and was sitting on the bed, quite jolly, drumming with his stumps.

A poignant image that wouldn't be out of place in a Dickens novel. Dr. Wollaston did his best to establish the cause of this unusual complaint, but eventually had to admit defeat. A local clergyman with a bleakly appropriate name, the Reverend Mr. Bones, offered to make further inquiries. He questioned the family minutely about where they bought their food and drink, and even examined their cooking implements. But he, too, drew a blank:

---

* Gangrenous

I have taken all the pains I can to inform myself of every cir-cumstance which may be deemed a probable cause of the dis-ease, by which the poor family in my parish has been afflicted. But I fear I have discovered nothing that will be satisfactory to you.

John Downing himself attributed his family's misfortune to witch-craft, a suggestion that the priest naturally discounted. Dr. Wol-laston came closest to solving the problem when he made this observation:

The corn with which they made their bread was certainly very bad: it was wheat, that had been cut in a rainy season, and had lain on the ground till many of the grains were black and to-tally decayed; but many other poor families in the same village made use of the same corn without receiving any injury from it.

An editor at the *Philosophical Transactions* then made a connec-tion that Dr. Wollaston had missed: Half a century earlier, a French surgeon had noticed something strikingly similar. In an article published in 1719, Monsieur Noël, a surgeon from Orléans, wrote that he . . .

. . . had received into the hospital more than fifty patients af-flicted with a dry, black and livid gangrene which began at the toes, and advanced more or less, being sometimes continued even to the thigh.

This aroused great interest when M. Nöel presented his findings to the members of the French Royal Academy of Sciences.

*The gentlemen of the academy were of opinion, that the disease
was produced by bad nourishment, particularly by bread, in
which there was a great quantity of ergot.*

Hitting the nail right on the head. Ergot is grain that has been infected by a parasitic fungus, *Claviceps purpurea*. The tainted grain takes on a dark blue-black hue and contains toxic chemicals that are unaffected by heat, so baked foodstuffs such as bread are still dangerous to eat. The toxins can even be passed from mother to child via breast milk, which explains the death of John Downing's infant son. Dr. Wollaston's article is a classic description of the symptoms of gangrenous ergot poisoning.

In October 1762, six months after his first visit, Dr. Wollaston returned to John Downing's house. He was pleased to find that John's wife, Mary, was still alive:

*In my former account . . . I mentioned that one of her feet had
separated at the ankle, and that the other leg was perfectly
sphacelated to within a few inches of the knee, but not then
taken off. Some little time afterwards the husband broke off the
tibia, which was quite decayed, about three inches below the
knee: the fibula was not decayed, so the surgeon sawed it off.*

Cases of ergotism are still encountered from time to time, but, thankfully, such scenes of horror are long gone.

THE HUMAN PINCUSHION

In 1825, a doctor from Copenhagen published a case so incredible that he felt it necessary to point out that thirty of his colleagues could corroborate the story. Dr. Otto's article appeared originally in a German journal, but the editors of the *Medico-Chirurgical Review* then translated it for the benefit of an English-speaking audience:

14. THE COPENHAGEN NEEDLE PATIENT.

Rachel Hertz had lived in the enjoyment of good health up to her fourteenth year; she was then of a fair complexion, and rather of the sanguineous temperament.

At this period many physicians still believed in four "temperaments," or personality types. This was a relic of the ancient idea of the four humors, which had dominated medicine at least since the era of Hippocrates in the fourth century BC. According to humoral theory, disease was caused by imbalance among four bodily fluids, or humors (blood, phlegm, yellow bile and black bile). The "sanguineous" temperament was associated with an abundance of blood; one early-nineteenth-century doctor wrote that "people of this temperament are usually very strong, and all their functions are extremely active."

In August 1807, she was seized with a violent attack of colic, which induced her to apply to Professor Hecholdt, and this was the first acquaintance which the Professor had with the case. From that time to March 1808 she experienced frequent attacks of erysipelas* and fever, which left her in a very debilitated state. Many symptoms of an hysterical character showed themselves, but which the ordinary remedies failed to remove. From March to May 1809, a period of fourteen months, she

---

* A bacterial skin infection

suffered in this way from repeated and violent hysteric attacks,
accompanied with, or rather followed by, fainting, which
sometimes continued so long that people considered her dead.
Occasionally she was attacked with epileptic fits, at other times
with drowsiness and hiccough, and sometimes with delirium.

The next development says a lot about the leisure habits of edu-
cated Danish teenagers in the early nineteenth century. I don't suppose many modern patients are troubled by this symptom:

> *During the paroxysms of her madness, she delivered, with a*
> *loud voice and correct enunciation, long passages from the*
> *works of Goethe, Schiller, Shakespeare, and Oehlenschläger,*
> *just as accurately as any sane person could do, and although*
> *she kept her eyes closed, she accompanied the declamation with*
> *suitable gesticulations.*

Another journal, in its report of this case, included "long fits of
theatrical recitations from tragic poets" in its description. The association between Romantic literature and mental illness was quite
genuine: After the publication of *The Sorrows of Young Werther* in
1774, young men started to dress like Goethe's tragic hero and even
emulate his melancholic behavior, causing such alarm at the possibility of copycat suicides that several countries banned the book.
There is no suggestion, however, that this was what ailed poor Rachel Hertz:

> *The delirium continued to increase until it assumed a very*
> *alarming height; she gnashed her teeth, kicked about, and*
> *fought with whatever came in her reach, and disturbed with*

*her ravings, not only her own household, but the whole neigh-
bourhood.*

The girl's obvious mental distress was now compounded by physical ailments: Constipation and difficulty in urinating necessitated
the daily use of a catheter. Most seriously, she began to vomit blood.
The fits of mania began to retreat, and she sank into a stupor from
which, apparently, nothing would rouse her.

*In May 1809, Professor Collisen was consulted, who during the
lethargic state of the patient recommended snuff to be pushed
up her nostrils, the effect of which was so favourable that, without sneezing, she soon came to her senses. She complained of
nothing during that day, and the snuff frequently produced
equally good effects, for a time only. The delirium continued
from May 1809 to December 1810, with little variation of importance, and then gradually subsided.*

She remained in much better health for the next few years, apart
from one brief relapse. Until January 1819, when

*severe colic pains made their appearance, with fever, vomiting of
blood, and purging of black faecal matter, from which it was
considered impossible that she could recover—but recover she
did. On examination of the abdomen, a large tumour was
found, having three distinct elevations just below the umbilicus.*

Soothing dressings were placed on this swelling, but to no avail. In
desperation, Professor Hecholdt decided to open the tumor with
the scalpel. And this is where things started to get *really* interesting.

It was expected that a copious discharge of pus would follow, but no pus came, and the bleeding was very slight. When the wound was examined with a probe, a curious sensation was communicated to the hand, just as if a metallic body had been thrust against the probe; this was repeated, a forceps was introduced, the substance was laid hold of, and, to his great astonishment, out came a needle. The extraction of this needle produced some alleviation of the sufferings of the patient, but it was of very short duration; great pain with vomiting of blood returned, another tumour appeared in the left lumbar region, the touching of which caused great uneasiness. On the 15th of February, an incision was made into it, and another black oxidised needle drawn out.

Similar lumps started to emerge all over the young woman's body. Each time one appeared, the doctors cut it open, always with the same result:

From the 12th of February 1819, to the 10th of August 1820, a period of eighteen months, severe pains, followed by tumours, were felt in various parts of the body, from which two hundred and ninety-five needles were extracted, viz.—
From the left breast, 22; from the right breast, 14; from the epigastric region, 41; from the left hypochondriac region, 19; from the right hypochondriac region, 20; from the umbilicus, 31; from the left lumbar region, 39; from the right lumbar region, 17; from the hypogastric region, 14; from the right iliac region, 23; from the left iliac region, 27; from the left thigh, 3; from the right shoulder, 23; between the shoulders, 1; from under the left shoulder, 1.
Total—295.

Between August 1820 and March 1821, no further needles appeared; assuming his patient was cured, Professor Hecholdt wrote a pamphlet (in Latin, naturally) documenting the strange facts of the case. But this turned out to be premature:

> *A large tumour formed in the right axilla,* from which, between the 26th of May and the 10th of July, 1822, no less than one hundred needles were taken out! From the 1st of July, 1822, to the 10th of December, 1823, five needles were at different times extracted, making the total number of FOUR HUNDRED!!*

The emphasis is in the original; the author could barely contain his excitement.

> *The patient has amused herself during her convalescence by learning Latin, and writing a journal of her own case. She is at present living at Frederick's hospital, at Copenhagen, and enjoys good health.*

Oddly, the article in the *Medico-Chirurgical Review* does not attempt to explain the emergence of several hundred needles from different parts of the patient's body. Incredible as it may seem, the most likely explanation is that she had swallowed them. She probably had an eating disorder called pica, in which the patient compulsively ingests inedible objects such as soil or paper. Once inside the body, needles have a nasty habit of piercing the walls of the digestive tract and then migrating all over the body. This would explain the girl's stomachaches, her vomiting of blood, and finally the dramatic appearance of rusty needles everywhere from her armpits

---

* Armpit

to her thighs. Not until the era of punk would so many dodgy piercings again be seen on a single human body.

THE MAN WHO FOUGHT A DUEL IN HIS SLEEP

If you've ever shared a house with a habitual sleepwalker, you may be familiar with the strange experience of having a conversation at 2 A.M. with somebody who is fast asleep. One of my sisters went through a sleepwalking phase in childhood, and we soon became used to guiding her back to her bedroom, while saving the weirdest of her utterances for gleeful quotation at breakfast the next morning.

But as somnambulists go, it turns out that she was a mere amateur. In 1816, a London medical journal told the story of a Dutch student identified only as Mr. D.:

> AUTHENTICATED CASES,
> OBSERVATIONS, AND DISSECTIONS.
> XL.—*A singular Case of Somnambulism.*

In 1801, young Mr. D. went to stay as a paying guest at the home of the Reverend Mr. H., a respectable priest with a young family. On his arrival he warned his hosts that he sometimes walked in his sleep; they were not to be alarmed if he did so. A few nights later the clergyman was woken by an unusual noise, and went downstairs to investigate:

I found Mr D. in his sleep taking down some of his books, which had been sent him by his parents. I stayed in the room some time, not choosing to wake him on the sudden. On further examination, I perceived he was employed in making a catalogue of them quite in the dark, and with as much precision as I could have done with a light; making no mistakes with regard to the titles of the books, the names of their authors, their respective editions, and where they were printed. On letting one of the books fall, the noise appeared to have startled him, and he hastily retired to bed.

The next morning, the young man had no memory of the incident. He was capable of surprisingly elaborate tasks while asleep: He played chess and cards, and once wrote a letter to his professors— in Latin.

At another time, when he was to deliver a Latin oration in public, we heard him in his somnambulant state rehearse it aloud, as though the curators of the school were present; and as he was feeling for the desk to lay his thesis upon, Mr H. stooping a little before him, he laid it upon his neck, supposing it to be the rostrum. When he had finished his oration, he bowed to the audience and to the curators, as if present, and then retired.

On another occasion after he had gone to bed, the landlord's daughter began to play the piano. Mr. D. arrived in the room with a score, pointed to a favorite piece and placed it on the music stand for her to play. When she had done so, Mr. D. and the family all applauded. He then left the room hurriedly, having apparently just woken up and realized that he was undressed.* For the most part, his behavior when asleep was calm and rational, although there was one notable occasion when this was not the case:

He supposed one night that he must fight a duel with one of his former fellow-students at Utrecht, and asked Mr H. to be his

---

* Most of us have had the oh-God-I'm-naked-and-everybody-else-has-their-clothes-on anxiety dream. Imagine it happening for real! The horror.

second; the hour was fixed, the ground measured, and when the signal was given, down fell Mr D. as mortally wounded, and requested to be put to bed, and a surgeon to be sent for immediately. As a surgeon of our acquaintance desired to see him in his somnambulant state, we sent for him. When he asked Mr D. where he was wounded, he put his hand to his left side, saying "here, here— here is the ball." "I am come to extract it," said the surgeon; "but before I begin the operation, you must take some of these drops which I have brought with me." After that, making some great pressure upon the side where Mr D. said he was wounded, the surgeon said the ball was out. Mr D. felt at his side— "so it is," he said; "I thank you for your skilful operation. Is my antagonist dead?" he asked; and when they told him he was living, joy beamed in his countenance; and it appeared as if that joy awakened him.

Quite a yarn. The editor of *The London Medical Repository* evidently feared it might be thought a bit *too* good, since he appended to it this wry little footnote:

This letter was put into our hands by a practitioner of great respectability, with the assurance that he could vouch for the authenticity of the facts it details, being personally acquainted with the writer, who is a clergyman in Holland of high character and undoubted veracity. The facts are of so very singular a description, that, notwithstanding the source from which they proceed, we conceive it proper to give them to our readers accompanied by this testimony: we leave them to the degree of credence to which they may be considered entitled.

Quite.

THE MYSTERY OF THE EXPLODING TEETH

This engaging little mystery first appeared in the pages of *Dental Cosmos*—the first American scholarly journal for dentists, founded in 1859. I love the title; imagine going into your local store and asking for "a pint of milk and *Dental Cosmos*, please." In one of its early issues, W. H. Atkinson, a dentist from Pennsylvania, wrote to the journal to report three strange and similar cases that he had encountered over a period of forty years in practice.

EXPLOSION OF TEETH WITH AUDIBLE REPORT.
BY W. H. ATKINSON.

The first of his subjects was the Reverend D.A., who lived in Springfield in Mercer County, Pennsylvania. In the summer of 1817, he suddenly developed an excruciating toothache.

> *At nine o'clock a.m. of August 31st, the right superior canine or first bicuspid commenced aching, increasing in intensity to such a degree as to set him wild. During his agonies he ran about here and there, in the vain endeavor to obtain some respite; at one time boring his head on the ground like an enraged animal, at another poking it under the corner of the fence, and again going to the spring and plunging his head to the bottom in the cold water; which so alarmed his family that they led him to the cabin and did all in their power to compose him.*

This is not terribly dignified behavior for a clergyman. That toothache must have hurt *a lot*.

*But all proved unavailing till at nine o'clock the next morning,
as he was walking the floor in wild delirium, all at once a
sharp crack, like a pistol shot, bursting his tooth to fragments,
gave him instant relief. At this moment he turned to his wife,
and said, "My pain is all gone."*

To be fair, so was his tooth.

*He went to bed, and slept soundly all that day and most of the
succeeding night; after which he was rational and well. He is
living at this present time, and has vivid recollection of the dis-
tressing incident.*

The second case took place thirteen years later; the sufferer
this time was a Mrs. Letitia D., from Mercer County in Pennsylvania:

*This case cannot be so clearly or fully traced as case first, but
was much like it, terminating by bursting with report, giving
immediate relief. The tooth subsequently crumbled to pieces; it
was a superior molar.*

A final example occurred in 1855, also in Mercer County (was it
something in the water?), the victim a Mrs. Anna P.A.:

*This had a simple antero-posterior split, caused by the intense
pain and pressure of the inflamed pulp. A sudden, sharp report, and instant relief, as in the other cases, occurred in the
left superior canine. She is living and healthy, the mother of a
family of fine girls.*

Though it's good to know that she's well and has a family, I doubt many readers would have been expecting a minor dental incident to be life-threatening.

Dr. Atkinson's report seems to have presaged a mini epidemic of detonating dentine, as a number of similar cases came to light over the next couple of decades. In a book published in 1874, *Pathology and Therapeutics of Dentistry*, J. Phelps Hibler described one particularly striking example. His patient was a woman whose tooth was aching so badly that she felt she was losing her wits:

> *All of a sudden the raving pains eased up greatly; having been walking the floor for several hours, she sat down a moment or two to take some rest. She averred that she had all her senses unimpaired from the moment aching ceased; all at once without any symptom other than the previous severe aching, the tooth, a right lower first molar, burst with a concussion and report that well-nigh knocked her over.*

The tooth was split through from top to bottom, the impact of the explosion "rendering her quite deaf for a considerable length of time." It was as if a firecracker had gone off inside her mouth.

If we are to believe such accounts, these were quite dramatic explosions. So what might have caused them? In his original article, Dr. Atkinson suggested that a substance that he called "free caloric" was building up inside the tooth and causing a dramatic increase of pressure. This hypothesis can be ruled out straight away, since it relies on an obsolete scientific theory. For many years, heat was believed to consist of a fluid called caloric, which was self-repelling—although this would make a pressure increase plausible, we now know that no such fluid exists. J. Phelps Hibler had a different idea: He believed that caries (tooth decay) inside the dental pulp generated flammable gases that eventually exploded. But this is no more plausible, since we now know that caries is a process that starts on the *outside* of the tooth, not its interior.

Several other theories have since been proposed and rejected, ranging from the chemicals used in early fillings to a buildup of electrical charge. The most likely explanation seems to be that the patients were exaggerating symptoms that were far more mundane. Teeth do sometimes split if you bite into something hard, and the noise it makes can seem quite dramatic if it's inside your own jaw. But even this fails to explain the "audible report" claimed by several witnesses; like the fate of the *Mary Celeste*, or the identity of Jack the Ripper, all remains shrouded in obscurity. For now, at least, it seems that the mystery of the exploding teeth will remain unsolved.

THE WOMAN WHO PEED THROUGH HER NOSE

Dr. Salmon Augustus Arnold, an obscure general practitioner from Providence, Rhode Island, has not left much of a mark on history. He does have one claim to immortality, however: a perplexing report that he provided for *The New England Journal of Medicine and Surgery* in 1825. It reads like a Rabelaisian version of *The Exorcist*, complete with horrifying plot twists and inexplicable bodily fluids. Dr. Arnold believed he had identified a rare illness new to science, which he called *paruria erratica*—a Latin phrase meaning "wandering disorder of urination." A strange name, but curiously apt:

Case of Paruria Erratica, or Uroplania. By SALMON AUGUSTUS ARNOLD, M.D.

Maria Burton, aged 27 years, of sound constitution, generally enjoyed good health until June 1820, when she was afflicted with a suppression of the catamenia accompanied with haemoptysis.

Translated into English: She had missed her period and was spitting blood.

The physicians in attendance, irregular practitioners, bled her profusely every other day, and after the system had become greatly debilitated, injudiciously administered emetics, the operation of the last of which was succeeded by a prolapsus uteri, and a total inability to perform the function of urinary secretion. In this state she continued for nearly two years and a half without any alleviation of the disease, though for the most part of the time under the care of respectable physicians.

A prolapsed uterus occurs when the muscles and ligaments holding it in position in the abdomen weaken and stretch. The organ then slips down into the vagina. A common complication of the condition is a prolapsed bladder, causing inability to urinate, which is clearly what had happened in this case. It was now necessary to insert a catheter into her bladder once a day to draw off the urine. This is where things started to turn very . . . weird.

In September 1822, soon after I first saw her, the urine not having been drawn off by the catheter for seventy-two hours, found an outlet by the right ear, oozing drop by drop, and continued for several hours after the bladder had been emptied. The next day at five o'clock pm it again commenced and continued about as long as on the day preceding, but a larger quantity was discharged. This was thrown on to a heated shovel, and gave out the odor so peculiar to urine, indicating the presence of urea.

The "heated shovel test" is inexplicably no longer a part of conventional diagnostic practice. The discharge of urine from the ears continued, becoming more frequent each day. It was, reports Dr. Arnold,

increasing gradually in quantity, and being discharged in less time, until a pint was discharged in fifteen minutes in a stream about the size of a crow quill; then becoming more irregular, being discharged every few hours, and increasing in quantity, until eighty ounces were discharged in twenty-four hours.

That's four pints, more than the average person urinates in a day. New symptoms then appeared: She started to suffer from spasms and "swooning." At times she would laugh, sing and talk incoherently, though "frequently with an unusual degree of wit and humor"; at others she remained catatonic for up to twelve hours. And worse was to come.

The sight of the right eye was soon destroyed, and frequently that of the left was so impaired that she could not distinguish any object across the room, but the latter is now entirely restored. The hearing of the right ear is so much impaired that

she cannot distinguish sounds, and there is a constant confused
noise heard by her like the roaring of a distant waterfall.

Strangely, this imaginary waterfall soon turned into the real thing:

The next outlet the urine found was by the left ear, a few mo-
ments previous to which discharge, a similar noise is heard to
that noticed in the right ear: she cannot hear distinctly for ten
or fifteen minutes previously, and after the urine passes off.
Soon after the discharge from the left ear, the urine found an-
other outlet by the left eye, which commenced weeping in the
morning and continued for several hours, producing consider-
able inflammation.

Look, this is getting ridiculous. But wait, there's more.

On the 10th of March, 1823, urine began to be discharged in
great quantities from the stomach, unmixed with its contents.
On the 21st of April, the right breast became tense and swollen,
with considerable pain, and evidently contained a fluid, a few
drops of which oozed from the nipple. Urine has been dis-
charged occasionally from the left breast.

So far, we have urine coming from both ears, both eyes, the stomach and both breasts. There can't be any more orifices left, surely?
There can:

May 10th, 1823: the abdomen about the hypogastric and um-
bilical region became violently and spasmodically contracted
into hard bunches, and a sharp pain was felt shooting up from
the bladder to the umbilicus, around which there was a severe

twisting pain; in a few days subsequently a loud noise was heard, similar to that produced by drawing a cork from a bottle, and immediately afterwards urine spirted out from the navel, as from a fountain.

The poor woman's experience sounds pretty ghastly, but you have to admit that a fountain of urine gushing from her navel must have been quite a sight. Incredibly, the *pièce de résistance* was yet to come:

Nature wearied in her irregularities, made her last effort, which completed the phenomena of this case, and established a discharge of urine from the nose. This discharge commenced on the 30th of July, 1823, oozing in the morning guttatim* and increasing in quantity every day until it ran off in a considerable stream.

Was the liquid really urine? Dr. Arnold sent several samples to a professor of chemistry, who analyzed them and confirmed that they contained a high proportion of urea, an organic waste product found in normal urine. The next obvious question: Was this phenomenon genuine, or was the woman faking it somehow?

To remove every doubt, I and my friend Dr. Webb, who at my request had occasionally attended her, remained with her four hours alternately, during twenty-four hours, and the quantity discharged during this time was as large as it had been for several days previous to, and after this period. There has never been any doubt that these fluids, which have been proved to be

---

* Drop by drop

urine, were actually discharged from the ear and the other out-
lets, since the fact has been proved, day after day, by ocular
demonstration.

The doctor could have written "I saw it myself" but decided that
the gratuitously highfalutin "by ocular demonstration" sounded
better. So what happened to her? The story has a happy ending—of
a sort:

This great disturbance in the system continued to increase for
nearly six months, and it was the opinion of all who saw the
patient that she could not survive from day to day; after which
period it gradually abated, and she is now, when the urine is
freely discharged, so much relieved that she is able to walk
about her room, and during the summer of 1824 frequently
rode out. The discharges from the right ear, the right breast
and navel continue daily, but they are not so great nor so fre-
quent as they were a year since; from the bladder the quantity
is as usual; from the stomach, nose, eye, there has for some
months been no discharge.

Not ideal: A tendency to urinate spontaneously from the ear does
not make one the perfect dinner-party guest. The report concludes
with what Dr. Arnold calls a "diary of the discharges": a heroic,
seventeen-page document recording how much urine the patient
produced each day over a nine-month period, as well as the ori-
fice(s) from which it emerged.

If you're thinking the whole thing sounds too far-fetched to be
true, you're probably right. But there is just the faintest chance
that Maria Burton was suffering from an exotic combination of
conditions with bizarre symptoms. We know that her illness began

with a prolapsed uterus, which caused an obstruction to the urinary tract. If the body can't get rid of its waste products in the urine, the blood can become saturated with urea, a condition known as uremia. Typical symptoms include fatigue, abnormal mental state and tremors, all of which were present in this case. But the most striking feature of uremia, seen only in patients with kidney failure, is uremic frost, in which urea passes through the skin and crystallizes. When dissolved in sweat, it produces a liquid that smells and looks like urine. And if she was suffering also from edema—a buildup of fluid in the tissues—this smelly perspiration might have been quite copious.

Ah, but what of the urine that "spirted out from the navel, as from a fountain"? Astonishingly, there may be a rational explanation for that, too. The bladder is connected to the navel by a structure called the urachus, the vestigial remnant of a channel that drains urine from the fetal bladder during the early months of pregnancy. This tube usually disappears before birth, leaving just a fibrous cord, but very occasionally it persists into later life.* When the channel is very narrow, it may not be noticed, but if pressure builds up in the bladder, urine can be forced through the opening and out through the belly button.

Case closed? Not exactly. A patient with such severe uremia would be lucky to survive for six months, let alone two years. And that's not the only problem. It is not just unlikely but physiologically impossible for urine to be discharged from the ear, or from the nose for that matter.† Either Maria Burton was the only person in medical history to have peed through her nose or she

* A condition known as patent urachus
† Hilariously, several old medical dictionaries include the word *oturia*, defined as "urine discharged from the ear"—a word for a phenomenon that does not (and cannot) occur.

was very good at faking it. And I know which of the two is more likely.

THE BOY WHO VOMITED HIS OWN TWIN

This delightful case was originally reported in a Greek newspaper in 1834, and quickly caused a sensation in the European medical press. Pierre Ardoin, a French doctor who had settled on the Aegean island of Syros, was summoned by the worried parents of a young boy called Demetrius Stamatelli who had fallen ill. This is how one London journal reported the tale:

> ### ABORTION EXTRAORDINARY.
> #### FŒTUS VOMITED BY A BOY.

On the 19th July last, when M. Ardoin was called to see this youth, he found him suffering from acute pains in the abdomen. He prescribed several remedies, none of which in the least assuaged his torments, and he so far gave up all hope of saving the patient that he recommended the administration of the sacrament.

Either Dr. Ardoin detected some signs of improvement or the parents took violent exception to his giving up on their son, because he soon decided that there were more useful things he could do for the boy than arrange the last rites.

The next day he gave him an emetic cathartic, which produced at first slight vomiting.

The "emetic cathartic" was a vile-sounding concoction of castor oil, coralline* and ipecacuanha.† Its effects would not have been pretty, since it was intended to provoke both vomiting and diarrhea.

This lasted a short time, when the vomiting returned with excessive pain, and at length he vomited a foetus by the mouth.

OK. He vomited . . . a fetus?

The head of the foetus was well developed, also one arm perfectly formed; it had no inferior extremities, but merely a fleshy prolongation, thin at the extremity, and attached to the placenta by a kind of umbilical cord. Three days afterwards the patient was much better, all the morbid symptoms were diminished, and he has since continued to improve.

Dr. Ardoin took the unexpected object home and invited all the other doctors of Syros to join him in examining it, after which it was preserved in alcohol. "I made it thus public," writes Dr. Ardoin, "so that it might not be considered a deception."

Sure enough, there were many who doubted the veracity of Dr. Ardoin's account. Members of the Academy of Sciences in Paris were suspicious of the "extreme zeal" with which he had publicized the case, and asked the distinguished naturalist Étienne Geoffroy Saint-Hilaire to investigate further. Saint-Hilaire had a particular interest in teratology, the study of congenital deformities, so was ideally qualified for this task. He arranged for the

---

* The dried leaves of a marine plant found in the Mediterranean
† The root of a South American plant then commonly used to treat dysentery

preserved fetus to be sent to him in Paris and, after dissecting it, pronounced himself satisfied that it was indeed a partially formed human fetus.

In the meantime, the young patient Demetrius Stamatelli had died, from causes unknown. The doctor who performed the autopsy found the boy's digestive tract virtually normal in appearance, and concluded:

The autopsy is far from confirming that he vomited a foetus; but neither does it prove that the story was made up, because of the time that had elapsed between the appearance of the foetus and the examination of the digestive organs.

There was, however, one intriguing anomaly: A small area of the stomach lining was unusually well supplied with blood vessels. A committee of medical experts in Athens agreed that this might have been the point at which the fetus was attached by its placenta. Saint-Hilaire's report took account of all these findings, concluding that although the case was far from proven, he could not rule it out entirely. He noted that if it *was* a hoax, the "simple and ignorant" parents of young Demetrius certainly had nothing to do with it.

As Saint-Hilaire knew, it is sometimes possible for one fetus to develop inside another, a phenomenon known as *fetus in fetu* (FIF). Demetrius may have shared his mother's womb with another fetus—his twin—which was subsequently absorbed into his own body. This is an incredibly rare occurrence, with fewer than two hundred cases recorded in the medical literature. In one extreme example, reported in 2017, a fifteen-year-old Malaysian boy was admitted to the hospital with abdominal swelling and severe pain; surgeons found a malformed fetus weighing 1.6 kilograms inside his body. What makes Demetrius's case unusual is the location of his "twin": Although FIF cases have been found inside the abdomen, skull, scrotum and even the mouth, it is difficult to believe that such an object could remain intact in the highly acidic environment of the human stomach for more than a few days.

THE CASE OF THE LUMINOUS PATIENTS

The Irish medic Sir Henry Marsh began his career hoping to become a surgeon, but at the age of twenty-eight he cut his forefinger while dissecting a cadaver and it became necessary to amputate the digit to prevent gangrene. His surgical ambitions thwarted, he instead became a physician, a profession in which he achieved great eminence. In 1821, he helped to found a children's hospital in Dublin—the first such institution in Great Britain and Ireland—and was later appointed a physician to Queen Victoria.

In an age when doctors were often imperious and forbidding, Marsh was known for his kindly and cheerful bedside manner. He was also renowned for the quality of his medical research on conditions including diabetes, fevers and jaundice. In June 1842, the *Provincial Medical Journal* devoted no less than ten pages to one of his essays. But what subject could be so important that a leading publication would make it the main feature of that week's issue? Sir Henry explains:

ON THE

EVOLUTION OF LIGHT

FROM

THE LIVING HUMAN SUBJECT.

By Sir HENRY MARSH, Bart., M.D.

Having obtained from an unquestionable and authentic source an account of a phenomenon of a very curious and interesting nature, not hitherto recorded or brought into public notice, I am induced to bring forward some facts I have been able to collect, illustrative of the spontaneous evolution of light from the living human subject.

That's right: Sir Henry's chosen subject is people who glow in the dark. It was his sincere belief that it is possible for the human body to produce its own light. Before unveiling his evidence for this startling assertion, however, he first points out that the phenomenon—known as bioluminescence—is quite common in marine organisms including plankton and deep-sea fish as well as a few insects such as fireflies.

Sir Henry reports a story told to him by a colleague who had attended the bedside of a young woman, identified only as L.A., who was dying from tuberculosis:

"It was ten days previous to L.A.'s death that I first observed a very extraordinary light, which seemed darting about the face, and illuminating all around her head, flashing very much like an Aurora Borealis."

An indoor northern lights is not quite what a doctor expects to see when tending a patient on their deathbed.

"After she settled for the night I lay down beside her, and it was then this luminous appearance suddenly commenced. Her maid was sitting up beside the bed, and I whispered to her to shade the light, as it would awaken Louisa. She told me the light was perfectly shaded. I then said, 'What can this light be

which is flashing on Miss Louisa's face?' The maid looked very mysterious, and informed me she had seen that light before, and it was from no candle."

A line that would not be out of place in a ghost story by M. R. James.

"I then inquired when she had perceived it; she said that morning, and it had dazzled her eyes, but she had said nothing about it, as ladies always considered servants superstitious. However, after watching it myself half an hour, I got up and saw that the candle was in a position from which this peculiar light could not have come, nor, indeed, was it like that sort of light; it was more silvery, like the reflection of moonlight on water."

Sir Henry did not witness the phenomenon himself but had it on good authority that one of his own patients was also affected. A few months earlier, he explains, he had been treating another young woman in the final stages of tuberculosis. Shortly after her death, he had received this intriguing communication from the girl's sister:

"About an hour and a half before my dear sister's death, we were struck by a luminous appearance proceeding from her head in a diagonal direction. The light was pale as the moon; but quite evident to mamma, myself, and sister, who were watching over her at the time. One of us at first thought it was lightning, till shortly after we fancied we perceived a sort of tremulous glimmer playing round the head of the bed; and then recollecting we had read something of a similar nature having been observed previous to dissolution, we had candles brought

into the room, fearing our dear sister would perceive it, and
that it might disturb the tranquillity of her last moments."

Sir Henry cites several other anecdotes of a similar nature, observing that in rural Ireland such occurrences were generally attributed to supernatural causes. As a man of science, he dismisses this as mere superstition, suggesting instead that as death approaches, some unidentified organic process may create phosphorescence around the human body. By way of illustration, he gives a final "luminous patient" story—this one supplied by Dr. William Stokes, an illustrious Dublin physician and one of the greatest heart specialists of the nineteenth century:

"When I was residing in the Old Meath Hospital, a poor
woman labouring under an enormous cancer of the breast was
admitted. The breast was much enlarged, and presented a vast
ulcer with irregular and everted edges, from all parts of which
a quantity of luminous fluid was constantly poured out."

Skeptical? For reasons that will be explained in due course, I believe Dr. Stokes may have been telling the truth.

"Upon being asked whether she suffered much pain, she an-
swered, 'Not now, Sir, but I cannot sleep watching this sore
which is on fire every night.' I directed that she should send for
me whenever she perceived the luminous appearance, and on
that night I was summoned between ten and eleven o'clock. The
lights in the ward having been then extinguished, she was
sitting leaning forward, the left hand supporting the tu-
mour, while with the right she every now and then lifted up the
covering of the ulcer to gaze on this, to her, supernatural

appearance. The whole of the base and edges of the cavity phos-phoresced in the strongest manner.

Dr. Stokes walked to the end of the ward and found to his amazement that he could still see the luminous tumor from a distance of twenty feet.

"The light within a few inches of the ulcer was sufficient to enable me to distinguish the figures on a watch dial. I have no very distinct recollection of the colour of the light, but I remember that its intensity was variable, it being on some nights much stronger than on others."

Sir Henry now attacks the most important question: What is the process responsible for this mysterious light? He speculates that when tissues begin to putrefy, they emit some luminous gas or fluid that is highly flammable. This would, he adds, explain the mystery of spontaneous human combustion: If the fluid were to ignite for some reason, perhaps the body itself could burst into flames. Sir Henry concluded that the luminescence observed in dying patients might have been caused by the presence of phosphorus, which burns spontaneously in the presence of oxygen. This theory is not tenable, because elemental phosphorus is far too reactive to be produced naturally by the human body. But there is one intriguing alternative.

In 1672, the natural philosopher Robert Boyle was thrilled to discover that a joint of veal hanging in his larder had started to glow in the dark. The luminous meat produced enough light to read by, of the same "fine greenish-blue as I have often observed in the tails of glow-worms." Boyle's joint had almost certainly been colonized by one of the many photobacteria, light-producing microorganisms found in seawater (and therefore in fish) all over the world. It has been known for years that poor food hygiene can result in cross-contamination if fish and meat are stored together; in a darkened room the surface of affected meat appears to be studded with points of light, like stars in the night sky. Most luminous bacteria are not human pathogens (agents of disease), but some are capable of colonizing the human body. If this is the case, it would offer one possible, albeit unlikely, explanation of the ghostly phenomena of Sir Henry's patients who glowed in the dark.

THE MISSING PEN

You know those stories about old soldiers who suddenly develop mysterious back pain in their eighties, and discover that it's caused by a bullet from their army days, long forgotten but still deeply embedded in tissue? They're usually true. Foreign objects made from all sorts of surprising materials are often well tolerated by the body and can lie dormant for decades before causing any problems.

Even in that context, this tale published in *The Medical Press and Circular* in 1888 is something of an outlier—not least because it concerns a foreign body that remained *in the brain* for as long as twenty years before symptoms became apparent.

AN EXTRAORDINARY INJURY.

The infliction of fatal injury to the brain by the thrusting of pointed objects beneath or through the upper eyelid, through the orbital plate into the brain, has occurred a number of times. Baby-farmers have been known to procure the death of their charges by pushing needles in.

"Baby farmers" were those who looked after another person's child
for money. Since they were often paid in one (small) lump sum,
many of them stood to profit if the child died. This led to many
cases of infanticide: After a campaign led by *The British Medical
Journal* in 1867, the law was reformed to introduce more rigorous
regulation of fostering and adoption.

*And not long since an irascible 'fare' thrust his stick some four
inches into the brain of a cab driver in the same way.*

I've sometimes been irritated by a cab driver, but I can't think of
circumstances in which this would be a proportionate response.

*The effect of such an injury is generally very prompt, and
within an hour or two—even if not at once—serious symptoms
manifest themselves. A curious exception to this rule was the
subject of an inquiry last week at the London Hospital, the victim being a commercial traveller 32 years of age. Until the last
few weeks the deceased is stated to have been in good health,
and to have kept a set of books most accurately.*

The patient is identified in contemporary newspaper reports as
Moses Raphael from Bromley-by-Bow in London's East End. Because of his facility with numbers, this peripatetic young gentleman was described as a "wonderful brain worker"—a somewhat
ironic description, as it turns out. Moses suddenly developed a
splitting headache and complained of drowsiness. He was admitted to the hospital and, a few days later, died after developing
symptoms of "apoplexy." This word was generally used to describe a cerebrovascular accident or stroke, but his doctors were in
for a shock:

On making a post-mortem examination of the brain, an abscess the size of a turkey's egg was discovered at the base, evidently not of recent formation, inside which was a penholder and nib, measuring altogether some three inches in length. This foreign body must have been in its position for some considerable time, it being embedded in bone. No trace of injury to the corresponding eye or nostril could be detected.

His widow was amazed: She had never heard him allude to anything of the kind, and nobody could recall his having been injured at any stage of his life.

The pen and nib were of the ordinary school pattern, and there is nothing to show that the injury was not inflicted years ago when the deceased was at school. Altogether, it is a very remarkable case and demonstrates the extreme tolerance of the brain to a very serious injury, and to the presence of a foreign body under certain circumstances. It is fortunate, in one sense, that the deceased died in a hospital; in private practice his death would have been certified as due to apoplexy, or, in case of an inquest, to 'visitation of God'.

"Visitation of God" was a verdict often returned in cases of sudden or unexplained death. In the case of this patient's demise, it seems unnecessary to invoke a deity—even one wielding a pen.

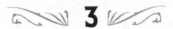

DUBIOUS REMEDIES

O NE THING MOST people know about the history of medicine is
that doctors used to prescribe some pretty strange courses of
treatment. For millennia, they were famously reliant on bleeding—
a therapy invented (at least according to the Renaissance scholar
Polydore Vergil) by the hippopotamus:

> *Of the water horse in Nylus, men learned to let blood: for when
> he is weak and distempered, he seeketh by the riverside the
> sharpest reed-stalks, and striketh a vein in his leg against it,
> with great violence, and so easeth his body by such means; and
> when he hath done, he covereth the wound with the mud.*

Some forms of bleeding were comparatively mild. Leeches, widely
used across Europe for hundreds of years, removed only a teaspoonful of blood per application. More drastic was venesection,
when the doctor opened a vein to evacuate larger volumes. The
technique was most often used on an arm, although it could be applied all over the body. In a treatise published in 1718, the German

surgeon Lorenz Heister gives instructions for taking blood from the eyes, the tongue and even the penis. One particularly enthusiastic exponent of bloodletting, the eighteenth-century American Benjamin Rush, encouraged his pupils "to bleed not only by ounces or in basins, but by pounds and by pailfuls." The practice finally died out in the nineteenth century, although a few older practitioners were still espousing it as late as the 1890s.

If you were lucky enough to escape a thorough bleeding, taking medicine often wasn't much fun either. Commonly prescribed drugs throughout this period included highly toxic compounds of mercury and arsenic, while naturally occurring poisons such as hemlock and deadly nightshade were also staples of the medicine cabinet. The *Pharmacopoeia Londinensis*, a catalogue of remedies first published in 1618, offers a fascinating insight into what used to be considered "medicinal" in seventeenth-century England. It includes eleven types of excrement, five of urine, fourteen of blood, as well as the saliva, sweat and fat of sundry animals. Other items you could routinely find in an apothecary's shop of the time included the penises of stags and bulls, frogs' lungs, castrated cats, ants and millipedes.

Perhaps the most bizarre items were discarded nail clippings (used to provoke vomiting), the skulls of those who had died a violent death (a treatment for epilepsy) and powdered mummy. The latter was prescribed for a variety of conditions including asthma, tuberculosis and bruising, and the premium stuff was imported from Egypt—although a cheap imitation could be prepared at home by dipping a joint of meat in alcohol and smoking it like a ham. Every bit as effective as the real thing, and a decidedly superior sandwich filling.

None of these odd remedies survived much beyond 1800, unsurprisingly, although all were perfectly orthodox in their day. As old medicines fell out of favor and new ones took their place, doctors frequently reported their experience with the new drugs in the professional journals. While some were deemed effective and gained general acceptance, others fell by the wayside. It is often the accounts of these failed remedies that make for the most entertaining reading—treatments that not only seem ridiculous today but were ridiculous from the moment they were conceived.

DEATH OF AN EARL

On a warm August afternoon, a man in his fifties is enjoying a game of bowls in the affluent English town of Tunbridge Wells. Suddenly he passes out and falls to the ground, apparently dead. If this scene were unfolding today, an ambulance would probably arrive in a few minutes, and paramedics would attempt resuscitation before whisking the poor man off to a hospital for urgent treatment. But what might have happened three hundred years ago? Thanks to an extraordinary document from the Bodleian Library in Oxford, reproduced in the *Provincial Medical and Surgical Journal* in 1846, we have a pretty good idea.

> ANECDOTA BODLEIANA: UNPUBLISHED
> FRAGMENTS FROM THE BODLEIAN.
> (*Continued from page* 44.)
> LETTER FROM DR. GOODALL TO SIR THOMAS
> MILLINGTON.

In 1702, the doctor Charles Goodall was staying with friends in Tunbridge Wells when his professional services were unexpectedly requested. Dr. Goodall, a celebrated medic who a few years later would be elected president of the Royal College of Physicians, described the tragic events in a letter to an eminent colleague, Sir Thomas Millington:

> *The most considerable accident which happened this season was the most sudden and surprising death of that great and eminent peer, the Earl of Kent, the true and full history of whose case is the following.*

The deceased was Anthony Grey, the 11th Earl of Kent, then aged fifty-seven.

> *His Lordship came very well to Tunbridge Wells, and continued so for about twelve days. He used no manner of exercise while he stayed, but only walking after morning prayers, for one hour or two, and sometimes after evening prayers, or on the bowling green at Mount Sion. On his Lordship's last and fatal day, I walked with him from the chapel two or three turns on the walks; he then made an appointment to meet at five in the evening to play at bowls, which he had not done before, nor drunk the waters during his continuance with us.*

In the early eighteenth century, most people who stayed at Tunbridge Wells were there to take the famous mineral waters. They were discovered—according to tradition—in 1606 by Dudley, Lord North, a dissipated young nobleman who recovered from a "lingering consumptive disorder" after drinking from a spring he had stumbled across in the woods. Dr. Goodall was himself at the spa for therapeutic reasons: His daily regime involved taking the waters and playing bowls for two hours every evening.

I went at the time appointed, and found my Lord on the green
before I got thither, engaged in bowls (if I mistake not), with the
Lord George Howard, Lord Kingsale, and Sir Thomas Powis.

A suitably aristocratic foursome.

I gave him an account of some news of which he had not
heard, which occasioned some discourse betwixt us; then he went
to his bowls, and played (I suppose) two or three games. I went to
the other end of the bowling green, and played one game and part
of a second, when on the sudden there was a cry, "A Lord is fallen!
A Lord is fallen! A surgeon! A surgeon!" upon which I left my
bowls, and ran up to his Lordship, and found him dead on the
ground, he having neither pulse nor breath, but only one or two
small rattlings in the throat, his eyes being closed.

"Neither pulse nor breath" seems pretty final: respiratory and cardiac arrest. Today any competent first-aider would administer
CPR, but this is a surprisingly modern technique, first described
as late as 1958. I at first assumed that an eighteenth-century medic
would realize the case was hopeless, but Dr. Goodall was not so
easily defeated.

He was bled immediately on both arms to the quantity of ten or
twelve ounces, as computed.

Slightly more than half a pint.

In the meantime I put up the strongest snuff and Spiritus Salis
Armoniaci into both nostrils, and ordered two ounces of Vinum

Benedictum to be brought with all speed. The apothecary (Mr
Thornton) sent for three ounces, which he poured down his
throat, not spilling one drop.

"Spiritus salis armoniaci" (sal ammoniac) is a solution of ammo-
nium chloride, an expectorant often used to treat chest complaints.
The highest-quality sal ammoniac came from Egypt and was manufactured from camels' urine. "Vinum benedictum" is antimonial
wine, wine adulterated with the toxic metal antimony and used as
an emetic. The doctor's plan, quite orthodox for the time, was to
shock the earl back to life by provoking an extreme reaction: sneezing, coughing or vomiting.

As soon as this was done we carried my Lord (in a chair) off the
bowling green through the dancing-room into a very sorry bed-
chamber, one pair of stairs. I supported his Lordship's head
(which otherwise would have fallen on one side, or backwards,
or forwards) with my hands and breast, till he was placed on a
bed in a little room; when this was done, I cried out for a sur-
geon to apply six or eight cupping glasses to his Lordship's
shoulders with deep scarification; but no surgeon or apothe-
cary (although one of the former and one of the latter were pres-
ent) had any, neither was there any to be had on the walks, (as
was answered by the surgeon or apothecary present), nor could
have been procured if the Queen's life had lain at stake on Tun-
bridge Wells.

Scarification with cupping was a mild form of bloodletting: Small
incisions were made in the skin, and the cupping glasses drew out
a modest volume of blood by suction.

When I found myself thus unhappily disappointed, I ordered his head to be shaved, and a large blister to be applied to capiti raso,* as also another to the breadth of neck and shoulders.

A blister was just what it sounds like: A harsh inflammatory substance was applied to the skin, usually on a plaster, in an attempt to provoke blistering and force toxins out of the body. The doctor also administered several spoonfuls of buckthorn syrup, a laxative. He was then joined by a colleague, one Dr. Branthwait, who had heard the news and hurried to offer his assistance. He suggested giving the dying man a "proper julep" (a refreshing infusion of herbs). The two medics certainly intended to be thorough. But the treatment was about to get rather more extreme:

Then Dr West came, who advised a frying pan made red hot to be applied to the head . . .

This sounds like desperation, and probably was.

. . . however there appeared not the least breath, pulse, or life in my Lord (though one or two physicians thought that there was some little umbrage† thereof), so that in short we had very slender hopes of his Lordship's case, or little or no encouragement from any application used.

At this point, Dr. Goodall became frustrated that the room was "crowded with lords and gentlemen," and asked them all to leave.

---

* His shaved head
† A glimmer or trace

One, the Bishop of Gloucester, went to break the news to the earl's
daughter, who lived a mile away.

> *She was (as must be imagined) upon the hearing of this news in
> a very great passion, crying out, "Is my Lord dead? is my Lord
> dead? tell me, my Lord, plain truth"; which being owned by the
> Bishop that his Lordship was dead, and of an apoplexy, she
> asked him whether cupping-glasses had been applied, and re-
> solved to go to her dear father.*

Distraught, the young woman asked for her father's body to be
brought back to his own apartment. Dr. Goodall agreed,

> *it being my judgment that the motion of the coach, with the
> warmth of my Lord's servant, who kept his body in an upright
> erect position by grasping him round the waist, might conduce
> to the operation of the vomit and purge which had been given
> him some hours before, if there was the least warmth or life left
> in his stomach or bowels, which might be so, though indiscern-
> ible to us.*

This was surely a forlorn hope: It sounds as if the poor man had
died within minutes of his original collapse. Nevertheless, the
earl's corpse (presumably) was propped up in a coach and taken to
his own lodgings. Even now the treatments continued:

> *As soon as his Lordship was put into his warm bed we ordered
> several pipes of tobacco thoroughly lighted to be blown up the
> anus, which we thought might be of use, when we could not
> have the advantage of tobacco glysters.*

A "glyster" is an enema. A liquid preparation of tobacco, which was known to be a stimulant, was routinely injected through the anus to treat a variety of conditions. On this occasion, however, they did not have any enema paraphernalia to hand, so instead resorted to blowing smoke up the dead man's bottom. Though this may sound an eccentric thing to do, it was a standard resuscitation technique, often employed in cases of drowning.* When even this failed to work, the doctors were at their wits' end. They tried one last desperate method, an attempt to warm the patient up:

After this was done, upon a suggestion of Sir Edmund King's, the bowels of a sheep killed in the house were applied to his Lordship's stomach and belly, but all without the least success, though we were reasonably encouraged to make use of all proper remedies in so great a case, many apoplecticks having come to life a considerable time after they appeared dead to all human sense.

An "apoplectick" is one who suffers apoplexy—what we would call a stroke or cerebrovascular accident (CVA). Stroke patients do indeed sometimes lapse into a coma and later recover, and three hundred years ago, medics often had great difficulty telling the difference between coma and death. Without a stethoscope, it was impossible to be absolutely sure that the heart had stopped beating; in some cases, it was safe to declare that death had occurred

---

* Those who administered the tobacco enema without due care and attention were liable to get a mouthful of the patient's rectal contents, a frightful possibility that made it a hazardous undertaking—not to mention an altruistic one. This is the origin of the expression "to blow smoke up someone's ass," meaning to behave in an ingratiating fashion. For more information on the delights of the tobacco enema, see the next case.

only once rigor mortis had set in. In that context, Dr. Goodall's perseverance in his resuscitation efforts is quite understandable.

The letter concludes with a lengthy discussion of the possible cause of death. Dr. Goodall's colleagues believed that the earl had died from an abscess or a "syncope"—the latter meaningless as a diagnosis, since it means simply "loss of consciousness." An abscess is also unlikely, since one could be expected to produce signs of infection before the patient's final collapse. There are in fact numerous things that might cause sudden death: a heart attack, cardiac arrhythmia or a burst aneurysm, for instance. But Dr. Goodall was strongly of the opinion that the fatal event had been a stroke, pointing out that when these are very severe

the patient is (as it was) planet-struck, or knocked down by a club, or butcher's axe, never more to move hand or foot after.

Just such a blow, he argued, felled the unfortunate Earl of Kent.

THE TOBACCO-SMOKE ENEMA

Samuel Auguste André David Tissot was an eminent Swiss physician of the eighteenth century, the author of one of the first scholarly studies of migraine, and also remembered for his much-cited work on the evils of masturbation, *L'Onanisme*. In 1761, he published *Avis au Peuple sur sa Santé*, a little book aimed at the general public and translated into English six years later.

One of the early readers of this work was John Wesley, the founder of Methodism, who was fascinated by medicine and even had a small practice as an amateur physician, giving free care to those who could not afford a proper doctor. In 1769, he published his own version of Tissot's work under the title *Advices with Respect to Health*. Although much of its guidance remains valid today, other sections are, well, a little outdated. Take, for instance, Tissot's advice on first aid in the event of near-drownings, which begins sensibly enough:

Directions with respect to drowned persons.

Whenever a person who has been drowned has remained a quarter of an hour underwater, there can be no considerable hopes of his recovery: the space of two or three minutes in such a situation being often sufficient to kill a man. Nevertheless, as several circumstances may happen to have continued life beyond the ordinary term, we should not give them up too soon, since it has often been known that after the expiration of two, and sometimes even of three hours, such bodies have recovered.

This sounds extremely unlikely. Seven minutes underwater is usually enough to cause fatal brain damage, and after half an hour, the chances of survival are virtually nil. Extremely cold water can increase this theoretical maximum, since hypothermia reduces the body's oxygen requirements and also triggers physiological mechanisms that effectively slow the metabolism. Even so, there are only a handful of cases in which people are known to have survived as long as an hour underwater, let alone two or three.

Tissot lists several measures that should be taken in order to improve the chances of recovery.

Immediately strip the sufferer; rub him strongly with dry coarse linen; put him as soon as possible into a well heated bed, and continue to rub him a considerable time together.

Before the advent of CPR, rubbing the body was thought to be the best way of restoring the circulation, even if the heart had stopped. Artificial respiration, on the other hand, was already known in the eighteenth century:

> *A strong and healthy person should force his own warm breath into the patient's lungs; and the smoke of tobacco, if some was at hand, by means of a pipe, introduced into the mouth.*

Imagine a paramedic giving mouth-to-mouth resuscitation while smoking a cigarette, and you'll get the general idea. Tissot, like many eighteenth-century doctors, believed that the primary cause of drowning was not necessarily inhaled water but the froth it created with gas inside the lungs. The theory behind this intervention was that tobacco smoke would dissolve this froth, causing the air to recover its "spring" or pressure—a technical term borrowed from the experimental writings of Robert Boyle. Bleeding was, naturally, another vital component of emergency treatment.

> *If a surgeon is at hand, he must open the jugular vein, and let out ten or twelve ounces of blood. Such a bleeding renews the circulation, and removes the obstruction of the head and lungs.*

And why stop at blowing tobacco smoke into the patient's lungs? Two orifices are better than one.

> *The fumes of tobacco should be thrown up, as speedily and plentifully as possible, into the intestines by the fundament. Two pipes may be well lighted and applied; the extremity of one is to be introduced into the fundament; and the other may be blown through into the lungs.*

Tissot even recommends using a pipe attached to a bladder for this purpose, much like the bag-mask ventilators used today by paramedics. Blowing tobacco smoke up the rectum was not some eccentric idea of his own: As we've already seen, the technique was employed in the failed attempt to revive the unfortunate Earl of Kent, and it was widely used in eighteenth-century Europe. It was known as Dutch fumigation, but the practice is believed to have been the invention of Native American tribes centuries earlier.

Tissot's book was published just before the emergence of the humane societies, organizations dedicated to the study and practice of resuscitation. The first of these, the Society for the Recovery of Drowned Persons, was founded in Amsterdam in 1767; others soon followed in Germany, Italy, Austria, France and London. Dutch fumigation was believed to be so valuable a technique that tubes and bellows for blowing tobacco smoke "into the fundament" were installed in public places such as coffee shops and barbershops—just as defibrillators are today. But it was not just smoke that might be used:

> Any other vapour may also be conveyed up, by introducing a cannula, or any other pipe, with a bladder firmly fixed to it. This bladder is fastened at its other end to a large tin funnel, under which tobacco is to be lighted. This contrivance has succeeded with me upon other occasions, in which necessity compelled me to apply it. The strongest volatiles should be applied to the patient's nostrils. The powder of some strong dry herb should be blown up his nose, such as marjoram, or very well dried tobacco.

It's a wonder the patient had any space left in his airways for oxygen, with all these substances being inserted into them.

As long as the patient shows no signs of life, he will be unable to swallow. But as soon as he discovers any motion, he should take within one hour, a strong infusion of carduus benedictus, of camomile flowers sweetened with honey; and supposing nothing else to be had, some warm water, with the addition of a little salt.

Carduus benedictus, also known as Holy Thistle, was believed to be a panacea by early modern medics: In *Much Ado about Nothing*, Margaret says to Beatrice: "Get you some of this distilled carduus benedictus and lay it to your heart; it is the only thing for a qualm."

Notwithstanding the sick discover tokens of life, we should not cease to continue our assistance since they sometimes expire after these first appearances of recovering. Lastly, though they should be manifestly reanimated, there sometimes remains an oppression, a coughing and feverishness; and then it becomes necessary sometimes to bleed them in the arms, and to give them barley-water plentifully.

The barley water doesn't sound too bad an idea, at least. Some of his suggestions are fairly dreadful, but Tissot concludes by condemning certain other treatments that are even worse:

These unhappy people are sometimes wrapped up in a sheep's, or calf's, or a dog's skin immediately flayed from the animal: but their operations are more slow, and less efficacious, than the heat of a well-warmed bed.

Yeuch. This was, in fact, a measure often resorted to—though more usually on the battlefield, where warm blankets were sometimes hard to come by.

The method of rolling them in an empty hogshead is dangerous
and misspends a deal of important time. That also of hanging
them up by the feet ought to be wholly discontinued.

Probably for the best. In fact, these were venerable and widespread
practices. The "hogshead" method entailed securing the patient on
top of (or within) a barrel placed on its side, which was then rolled
back and forth. This gentle oscillation was supposed to evacuate
water from the lungs, as was the cruder expedient of suspending the
patient upside down. But these techniques were already beginning
to go out of fashion: fifteen years later the influential Edinburgh
physician William Cullen denounced them, asserting that they were
"extremely dangerous, and often destroy the small remains of life."
Tissot concludes with another helpful tip:

The heat of a dung-heap may also be beneficial: and I have been
informed by a sensible spectator of it, that it effectually contributed
to restore life to a man, who had remained six hours under water.

I humbly submit that the "sensible spectator" was talking through
his fundament.

SALIVA AND CROW'S VOMIT

The University of Pavia in northern Italy is one of the oldest in the
world, founded in 1361. It has a distinguished history of experimental scientific research: Alessandro Volta, the pioneer of electro-
chemistry, was professor there for forty years beginning in 1779.

While Volta was working on his voltaic pile—the first electric
battery—his colleagues in the medical faculty were also producing

world-leading research. Alas, some of it has not aged well. An article in the *Annals of Medicine for the Year 1797* reports a lecture given by Dr. Valeriano Brera, a brilliant young physician who had been appointed professor at the tender age of twenty-two. In later years, Brera published a number of important works, including a book about parasitic worms that correctly challenged the theory, prevalent at the time, that such organisms were generated spontaneously inside the human body. But this earlier paper, reporting a clinical trial of a novel treatment that he had conducted in the city's hospital, is not quite in that class of scholarship:

Difcourfe on the Mode of Acting on the Human Body, by Means of Frictions made with Saliva and other Animal Fluids, and the various Subftances commonly given internally. Recited in the Hall of the Univerfity of Pavia. By Citizen Valerian Lewis Brera, M. D. Public Prof. Extraordinary of the Theory and Practice of Medicine; Clinical Lecturer, and Chief Surgeon to the National Legion of Pavia, &c. &c. Third Edition. 8vo. Pavia, 1ft of the Cif. Rep. (1797.)

This new method of exhibiting remedies, first proposed by Dr Chiarenti of Florence, and afterwards extended by Dr Brera of Pavia, has excited too much attention in Italy and in France, to permit us to leave it unnoticed, however little we may be disposed to coincide with its supporters in their opinion of its vast utility, and expectations of the benefits to be derived from it.

Not exactly a ringing editorial endorsement.

Dr Chiarenti recommended the gastric juice as an excellent remedy in diseases originating from debility of the stomach.

Making a patient ingest the stomach acid of another person (or animal, as it turns out) is certainly a brave clinical decision. The originator of the idea, Francesco Chiarenti, was a resourceful medical researcher who had published a book on the composition and function of stomach fluids.

In giving opium at the same time, he found that it often occasioned much uneasiness and vomiting. This he ascribed to its remaining on the stomach undigested, from the vitiated* gastric fluid not acting on it; and led him to reflect on the reasons why opium, administered externally, had so little action.

A question of huge interest to doctors of the late eighteenth century, particularly Italian ones. The anatomist Paolo Mascagni, who in 1787 published the first comprehensive description of the lymphatic system, had suggested that the quickest way of getting medicines into the circulation was not by swallowing them but through the skin. His doctrine, known as the iatroliptic† method, used ointments and unguents in place of oral medicines. But physicians who tried his method noticed that some drugs that were effective when ingested had almost no effect when rubbed on the skin. It was not at all clear why opium, for instance, was a powerful analgesic when swallowed but not when used as an ointment. Dr. Chiarenti

---

* Spoiled, corrupted
† From the Greek words *iatros* ("physician") and *aleiptes* ("anointer")

deduced that it was not absorbed in the stomach immediately but only after it had first been altered in some way by the gastric juices. If he could replicate this process outside the body, he reasoned, maybe it would be possible to make a preparation of opium that would pass through the barrier of the skin. He decided to test this theory by experiment.

An occasion soon offered. A woman, afflicted with violent pains, refusing to take opium by the mouth, was a fit subject for commencing his trials. He mixed three grains of pure opium with two scruples of the gastric juice of a crow.

Why a crow? This is not explained, but in his book, Dr. Chiarenti observes that crows are enthusiastic devourers of putrid meat, indicating that their gastric juices may be particularly powerful—if not necessarily the sort of thing you'd want to rub into your skin.

It soon emitted a strong and penetrating smell . . .

I bet it did.

. . . which diminished gradually. In half an hour, the opium was perfectly dissolved; but it was permitted to remain twenty-four hours. It was then mixed with simple ointment, and rubbed on the backs of the feet. In an hour, the pains were entirely gone; and, never returning, the woman remained cured.

This may have had nothing to do with the foul-smelling morphine/crow's vomit concoction, of course—faced with the prospect of a second dose, I would probably pronounce myself miraculously cured, too.

By the difficulty of procuring a sufficient quantity of the gastric fluid to enable him to carry his experiments the length he wished, he was led, by analogy, to substitute in its place saliva; and the result answered his expectations.

And why not? You may as well smear crow spit on your patients as crow vomit. Five other physicians tested the technique, using it to administer a variety of drugs, and claimed similar results. Professor Brera believed he had found what he was looking for: a way of turning an oral medicine into a topical ointment.

From all these observations, he is led to conclude, that every animalised fluid is fitted by nature to render remedies capable of being absorbed.

A number of Italian practitioners adopted Dr. Brera's methods with enthusiasm, and one or two eminent French physicians continued his research for a decade or so. But for some inexplicable reason, the crow's saliva ointment treatment never really caught on.

THE PIGEON'S-RUMP CURE

Eclampsia is a serious condition affecting women before, during or after childbirth. The name means literally "shining forth," a metaphor (or perhaps euphemism) for the seizures that characterize the condition, which arrive suddenly and dramatically. The cause of eclampsia has never been identified, although it is always preceded by pre-eclampsia—a combination of symptoms including high blood pressure and protein in the urine.

Until the late nineteenth century, doctors also recognized a malady they called the eclampsia of children. This was a misnomer: Although infants can suffer seizures that look like those observed in pregnant women, the likely causes of the two are quite different. For instance, infants affected by fever often display febrile convulsions, which look serious but do not necessarily indicate any sinister underlying condition.

In a textbook published in 1841, the *Handbuch der medizinischen Klinik* (*Handbook of the Medical Clinic*), the German physician Carl Friedrich Canstatt offered a really rather odd approach to treating children with "eclampsia":

> *One remedy I must mention here whose unequivocal effects I have myself witnessed, however inexplicable the phenomenon. If one holds the rump of a dove against the child's anus during paroxysm, the animal quickly dies and the attack ceases just as rapidly.*

One wonders what strange sequence of events led to this discovery. Ten years later, the *Journal für Kinderkrankheiten* (*Journal for Childhood Diseases*) picked up on this odd little aside. It reported that several physicians had been prompted to try the remedy for themselves. One of them was a Dr. Blik from Schwanebeck:

Ein sonderbares Mittel gegen die Eklampsie der Kinder.

> *A nine-month-old child, full-bodied, healthy and alert, with no signs of teething, was attacked by eclampsia, which recurred in ever-increasing seizures, and calomel,* valerian,† musk,‡*

---

* Mercury (I) chloride, a laxative
† An herb, often used as an antispasmodic
‡ A strong-smelling substance produced by the musk deer, also used as an antispasmodic

baths, mustard,* and enemas were used in vain. When yet another convulsion occurred, the anus of a young dove was held against the child's until the seizure was over. The attack was fierce, but the child survived.

Not long afterward, the journal received a communication from a reader in St. Petersburg. Dr. J. F. Weisse was the German-born director of the children's hospital in the Russian city:

> **Ein Beitrag zu Dr. Blik's Mittheilung über die Taubensteisskur gegen Eklampsie der Kinder; von Dr. J. F. Weisse zu St. Petersburg.**

Dr. Weisse had read the earlier article with interest. He was, he explained, already familiar with what later became known mockingly (in the English-language literature) as the "pigeon's-rump cure":

Long before the publication of Canstatt's Handbook I had already read—I do not remember where—about this strange method; but his approval induced me to apply it myself at an appropriate opportunity.

Dr. Weisse had, it transpires, used the magical pigeon's bottom on two separate occasions.

On August 13, 1850, during the night, I was called to a four-month-old child, who was suddenly attacked by eclampsia. After two days of unsuccessfully treating him by the usual means, and meanwhile believing this was a suitable opportunity for the

---

* Administered orally as an emetic, or in a poultice as a stimulant *experiment, on the third day I told the mother, a Russian lady of property, about this magical agent; I added, however, that I myself had little faith in it, but believed it to be completely harmless.*

Not having any faith in a treatment is not a terribly good starting point for using it, but I suppose if all else had failed, you can understand his position.

I had not been mistaken in my assumption, for the suggestion was met with approval, and they immediately proceeded to procure a pair of pigeons for the emergency. Early on the following morning, when I visited the little patient again and had almost forgotten the birds, I was received by the lady's fourteen-year-old son who opened the door, speaking to me in broken German: "The dove is dead and the child is very healthy; come on, Mama will tell you about it."

Certainly an arresting opening to a conversation.

The woman approached me with a joyful face, solemnly shook my hand and led me to her child, who was sleeping soundly. I learned that the previous day after my visit there had been several convulsions in quick succession, but at seven o'clock in the evening such a violent fit had occurred that, despairing of the boy's life, they had resorted to the pigeon. The woman's sister, who carried out the operation according to my instructions, told me that shortly after the bird had been applied to the child's anus it had gasped for air several times, closed its eyes periodically, then its feet had twitched in spasm and finally it had vomited. At the same time the child's seizures became weaker, until at the end of half an hour it sank into a peaceful sleep, which lasted for five hours. The pigeon, however, afterwards

could not stand on its feet, nor did it touch the food that had
been offered, and finally expired about midnight.

Net result: one healthy child, but one dead pigeon. You win some, you lose some. Dr. Weisse was encouraged by this experience but frustrated that he had not been on hand to witness the miraculous cure for himself. On the next occasion, he was more fortunate:

This case concerned a boy of one year and eight months who for
a long time had been suffering from dyspeptic disorders related
to dental work and had been under my medical supervision for
several weeks. On the evening of the 8th of October 1850 I re-
ceived a letter asking me to hurry as soon as possible to the
child, which had suddenly suffered a seizure.

When he arrived at the child's bedside, he found the boy unconscious, with trismus (a locked jaw) and half-closed eyes. Every so often, the child's face and extremities were gripped by spasms. The lockjaw made it impossible to give medicines by mouth, so the doctor suggested the pigeon cure:

A few minutes later a pair of pigeons was brought in and I was
able to put the procedure into practice myself. About ten min-
utes after the application, I noticed that the pigeon I was hold-
ing opened its beak several times, as if gasping for breath. The
child's spasms were now becoming more infrequent and weaker,
but his pulse was also sinking more and more. After half an
hour I realised that the pigeon had closed its eyes and let its
head hang down; it was dead. I now had the other animal
brought to me and laid it in the same way on the anus of the
child, whose pulse, however, could soon no longer be felt—and

after only ten minutes it lay there as a corpse. The dove, however, remained alive.

Scant consolation to the devastated parents. Dr. Weisse concludes with a mystifying appeal to his peers to continue this unusual research:

Finally, I cannot but urge all colleagues to repeat such experiments with the remedy as much as possible, for it seems clear what a great benefit to the treatment of children, especially those of the lower classes, would emerge if it were proved to happen this way.

Noting that St. Petersburg is teeming with pigeons, he also acknowledges that in other parts of the world, they are not so abundant. But he's got that covered, too:

In the meantime, experiments with other poultry are necessary.

You may think I'm being a bit hard on poor Dr. Weisse: After all, it's not fair to judge the doctors of two hundred years ago by today's standards. They had their reasons for choosing the remedies they used, however odd they may seem to the modern reader. But even many of his contemporaries thought Dr. Weisse's ideas were downright silly. An anonymous writer in the *British and Foreign Medico-Chirurgical Review* could barely withhold his glee, quoting Horace: "*risum teneatis?*" ("Can you help but laugh?") This is his pithy verdict on the treatment:

We mentally offered . . . the advice of an old French physician, who, on being asked his opinion of a new remedy that was highly praised for its extraordinary virtues in a certain disease, very gravely replied, "Dépêchez vous de vous en servir pendant qu'il guérit!"

The Frenchman's *bon mot* translates, more or less, as: "Hurry up and give it to him, while he's still getting better!"

MERCURY CIGARETTES

Nineteenth-century medical opinion on the subject of smoking was sharply divided. On the one hand, many prominent doctors condemned the practice as unhealthy, or even suggested that it caused cancers of the mouth; on the other, plenty of physicians believed that smoking eased coughs and other respiratory disorders by promoting the production of mucus. But for a brief period, some members of the profession also saw the cigarette as the ideal drug-delivery mechanism: Medications could be easily mixed with tobacco and then inhaled with the smoke. A definite step forward from the days of blowing it up the patient's bottom—although maybe not a very big step.

In 1851, the editor of the *London Journal of Medicine* gave his approval to an interesting new idea from the United States: cigarettes laced with mercury.

MATERIA MEDICA AND PHARMACY.

———

MERCURIAL INHALATION BY SMOKING CHEROOTS AND CIGARETTES.

The inhalation of various medicines along with the smoke of cigars or cheroots has been more than once recommended in this journal. In prescribing the method, the physician must take care that the patient be clearly told that the smoke is to be drawn into the lungs; and the mode of doing this must be properly explained to him.

Quite—suck all the health-giving carcinogens into those lungs!

Mr J.H. Richards, of Philadelphia, writes as follows in the Medical Examiner for June 1851—"I have been informed by a gentleman of intelligence, who has resided for a long time in China and Manilla, that mercury, which is there regarded as a specific in the severe forms of hepatic* disorder incident to the climate (and leading to its employment to an extent that would be considered extravagant by Europeans), is constantly exhibited in the following novel and peculiar manner. The black oxide† is introduced into the Manilla cheroots, and, being inhaled, is thus presented in the form of vapour to the most absorbent surface in the body.

An absolutely horrendous notion. When heated, the "black oxide" decomposes to metallic mercury, tiny droplets of which would have coated the mouth, airways and lungs.

"It certainly is a speedy plan of producing salivation. I mention this fact, as it is interesting in itself, and may suggest other applications of the same principle."

If you're going to kill yourself by smoking, you might as well do it even more quickly by smoking mercury, I suppose.

Would this plan be admissible in pneumonia? Perhaps not.

Given that pneumonia is a potentially fatal infection involving the lungs, "perhaps not" does not begin to cover it.

---

* Liver
† Mercury (I) oxide

It is right to state that the smoking of mercurialised cigars is by no means, as Mr Richards supposes, a novelty in the practice of medicine. The following formula was given many years ago by Bernard: "Cigarettes Mercurielles. Bichloride of mercury, 4 centigrammes; extract of opium, 2 centigrammes; tobacco deprived of its nicotine, 2 grammes." These cigarettes are recommended in syphilitic ulcerations of the throat, mouth, and nose.

Mercury, opium *and* tobacco! But that's just a glimpse of the possibilities. In 1863, the *Canada Lancet* gave a list of recipes for other "medicinal" cigarettes. In addition to the mercury cigarette, they recommended

Arsenical Cigarettes.

Yup, cigarettes containing arsenic, and made from blotting paper steeped in arsenous acid. The latter chemical is highly toxic and carcinogenic, and has been used to kill weeds, rats and mice. All things considered, smoking it is a Bad Idea.

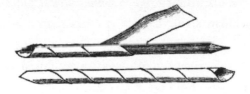

Nitre Cigarettes. Dip the paper in a saturated solution of the nitrate of potash before rolling.

Nitrate of potash, also known as saltpeter, is potassium nitrate, a component of gunpowder. Smoke with all due caution.

Balsamic Cigarettes are made by giving the dried nitre ciga-
rettes a coating of tincture of benzoin.

Tincture of benzoin is still sometimes inhaled in steam today, to ease
the symptoms of bronchitis, but . . . ! The article concludes with a list
of some of the miraculous cures attributed to medicated cigarettes:

Aphonia.—A patient who could not speak above a whisper for
over a year, probably due to a thickened condition of the chordae
vocales, as she had no pain or constitutional symptoms, used the
mercurial cigarettes for a month, and perfectly recovered.
Offensive discharges from the nostrils, with a sense of uneasi-
ness in the frontal sinuses, was quite cured in about a month
with the mercurial cigarettes. The patient held his nose after
taking a mouthful of the smoke, and then forced it into his nos-
trils in the manner practised by accomplished smokers.

Thus coating the delicate mucous membranes with fresh mercury
vapor.

Phthisis.—Trousseau long ago recommended a puff or two of
an arsenical cigarette twice or three times a day in phthisis.

Smoking while suffering from phthisis (tuberculosis) is perhaps the
very worst thing you could do. Especially if arsenic's involved.

When the attention of the profession has been duly aroused to
this subject, there will doubtless be found many other affections
in which medicated cigarettes may be advantageously employed.

No doubt. How about lung cancer?

THE TAPEWORM TRAP

In September 1856, an American journal, *The Medical and Surgical Reporter*, published a chatty "letter from New York." Their correspondent was a physician at one of the city's hospitals who called himself J. Gotham, Jr., MD. This was almost certainly a pseudonym: Although Gotham is best known as the fictional New York City of Batman and the Joker, the nickname first appeared in Washington Irving's periodical *Salmagundi* in 1807. Today, Gotham has noirish overtones, but for the nineteenth-century reader, the associations of the name were essentially farcical. Irving named his satirical version of New York after an English village whose residents had a reputation for idiotic behavior—a perfect analogy, he felt, for the incompetence of the municipal bigwigs who ran the city.

Dr. Gotham's dispatch from the cutting edge of New York medical science is certainly not short of absurdity:

A NEW AND ORIGINAL METHOD OF TREATING TAPEWORM.

As it is my desire to keep you advised of all the improvements in medical and surgical practice which this prolific age is ushering into being, it is my happy privilege now to bring to your notice one of the most ingenious, if not successful—the most far reaching, and deep searching, if not most likely to prove profitable, invention, ever accredited to Yankee wit and skill. It is one before which the lustre of the genius which produced the new operation for vaginal fistula must wax dim, and the discoverers of catheterism of the lungs must "pale their intellectual fires."

The "new operation for vaginal fistula" was devised by James Marion Sims in the 1840s, a surgical cure for an uncomfortable and embarrassing condition that often left women incontinent after childbirth.* "Catheterism of the lungs" was pioneered by the Vermont-born specialist Horace Green. It was a contentious treatment for tuberculosis that involved injecting silver nitrate directly into the lungs, using a rubber catheter passed down the patient's throat. Both these procedures were perceived as major advances, and emblematic of a new spirit of surgical adventure. As you've probably worked out, Dr. Gotham is drawing such comparisons ironically.

> *The government of the United States has immortalised its history by the issue of letters patent, securing to the inventor the exclusive right for fourteen years, of using a "Trap for Tapeworm", a description and engraving of which are given in vol. 1 for 1854 of the Patent Office Reports.*

The original patent for the tapeworm trap was filed by Alpheus Myers, a doctor from Logansport, Indiana. Dr. Myers was an exponent of Eclectic Medicine, a distinctly American school that rejected the chemical remedies and invasive procedures of conventional medicine. Instead of the poisonous laxatives and bloodletting favored by orthodox physicians, its adherents preferred plant remedies and gentle physical therapy. His invention was therefore an attempt to dispense with the toxic anthelmintic (anti-worm) agents then in use, such as powdered tin, calomel and even petroleum. Strangely, he patented not just the device but the operation for which it was

---

* Sims is a hugely controversial figure today, owing to the fact that he developed the procedure by performing experimental surgery on black slave women, possibly without informed consent.

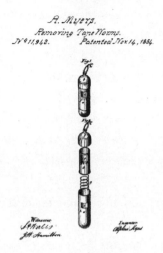

designed—thus ensuring that he would be the only person in the country allowed to use it. This is not a particularly clever thing to do if your aim is to sell your invention to lots of other people.

Another article from *The Medical and Surgical Reporter* describes the use of this unusual contraption:

> *The tapeworm trap is a very small hollow tube of gold so arranged as to contain a small piece of cheese for a bait. The patient, after a fast of four or five days, is ordered to swallow the trap, with a string attached. It is claimed by the inventor that after a long-continued fast, the worm comes up into the stomach, and will then greedily seize the cheese, be caught in the trap, and can be easily pulled out.*

This sounds most unlikely, not least because tapeworms live in the intestines and are averse to jaunts into the stomach, where the strongly acidic conditions would prove rapidly fatal. The inventor, Alpheus Myers, himself explains:

The cord is fastened to some conspicuous place about the patient, who is left to his ease from six to twelve hours, and during this time the worm will have seized the bait and have been caught by the head or neck. The capture of the worm will either be felt by the patient or ascertained by the motion which will be visible in the cord. The patient should rest for a few hours after the capture, and then by a gentle pulling at the cord the trap and worm will, with ease and perfect safety, be withdrawn.

The journal's correspondent comments, with not a little sarcasm:

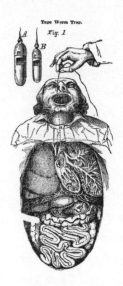

Imagine to yourself the satisfaction with which a man could thus sit down and fish in his own room, without even the accompanying tub of water; the patience and complacency with which, after waiting from six to twelve hours for a bite, he would then play his prisoner some hours more before landing him! Does not Mr Alpheus Myers have good reason to believe that the shade of Izaak Walton looks down upon him in anger for this innovation upon the piscatorial art?

Fishing for worms in one's own stomach does sound like a rather unappetizing way of spending an afternoon. In its coverage of the development, *Scientific American* claimed that "Dr. Myers, not long since, removed one fifty feet in length from a patient, who, since then, has had a new lease of life." A likely story.

Back to Dr. Gotham. His letter continues with a savage attack on the US patent office for even considering this nonsense:

My object in drawing the attention of your readers to it, is simply to expose the shameful ignorance, not of Alpheus Myers, but of the officers of our government, who would take money from a man for so gross an absurdity as this. There are physicians connected with the Patent Office, men whose names stand well before the country, and how they or the commissioner, could have allowed the seal of the office to be affixed to such a document for such a monstrously ridiculous contrivance, surpasses all comprehension.

He had a point. Not until 1965, when the husband-and-wife inventors George and Charlotte Blonsky succeeded in patenting their "Apparatus for facilitating the birth of a child by centrifugal force,"* would the US Patent Office rise to quite the same ludicrous heights.

THE PORT-WINE ENEMA

Alcoholic drinks were an important part of the physician's armory until surprisingly recently. In the early years of the twentieth century, brandy (or whiskey, in the US) was still being administered to patients as a stimulant after they had undergone major surgery. Every tipple you can think of—from weak ale to strong spirits—has been prescribed at one time or another.

But doctors didn't get their patients just to *drink* booze; indeed, they were remarkably imaginative in the strange things they did with it—injecting it into the abdominal cavity, for instance, or getting patients to inhale it. But this case, published in *The British Medical Journal* in 1858, trumps even those examples for sheer wrongheadedness.

---

* Seriously. Google it before you read the next story. You won't be disappointed.

PORT WINE ENEMATA AS A SUBSTITUTE FOR TRANSFUSION OF BLOOD IN CASES OF *POST PARTUM* HÆMORRHAGE.

No, you didn't misread the headline: This article seriously suggests a *port-wine enema* as an alternative to a blood transfusion. The author is Dr. Llewellyn Williams from St. Leonards-on-Sea in Sussex:

> *On September 22nd 1856 I was called into the country, a distance of four miles, to attend Mrs C., aged 42, then about to be confined of her tenth child. All her previous accouchements had been favourable. When about six months advanced in pregnancy, she received a violent shock by the sudden death of her youngest child, since which time her general health had become much impaired. She had a peculiar pasty anaemic appearance, and complained much of general weakness.*

Shortly after the doctor's arrival, a "fine female child" was born without much difficulty. But then:

> *My patient exclaimed, "I am flooding away," and fainted. I immediately had recourse to such restoratives as were at hand, and presently she began to revive.*

The poor woman's desperate shout was a literal description of her plight: She was bleeding heavily, at such a rate that she would soon be dead unless the hemorrhage could be arrested. Any improvement in her condition was short-lived, and Dr. Llewellyn Williams became seriously concerned.

> *My efforts still being foiled, and the haemorrhage continuing, the powers of life manifesting evident symptoms of flagging, I*

introduced my left hand into the uterus, after the manner recommended by Gooch,* endeavouring to compress the bleeding vessels with the knuckles of this hand, whilst with the other I pressed upon the uterine tumour from without. This combination of external and internal pressure was equally as unavailing as any of the other plans already tried. At last, by compressing the abdominal aorta, as recommended by Baudelocque the younger,† I was enabled effectually to restrain any further haemorrhage.

The abdominal aorta—the largest blood vessel in the lower half of the body—is only a few inches from the spinal column, so compressing it by hand is a procedure as difficult as it is drastic.

The condition of my patient had now become sufficiently alarming, she having been for upwards of half an hour quite pulseless at the wrist, the extremities cold, continual jactitation being present, the sphincters relaxed, and the whole surface bedewed with cold clammy perspiration.

Jactitation is pompous medic-speak for "tossing and turning." It was probably archaic even in the 1850s.

It now became a question what remedy could be had recourse to, which should rescue the patient from this alarming state, it being utterly impossible to administer any stimulant by the mouth. My distance from home, together with considerable

---

* Robert Gooch, an English physician and one of the leading obstetricians of the early nineteenth century. In 1821, he was the first to describe this method of arresting postpartum hemorrhage, which was widely adopted.
† Auguste César Baudelocque, nephew of the far more eminent Jean-Louis, the obstetrician who delivered Napoleon II

objections to the operation itself, which it is not here needful to
dwell upon, made me abandon the idea of transfusion of blood.

The first successful human blood transfusion was conducted by James Blundell in 1818, also for postpartum hemorrhage. But it was hideously risky: Blood types were not discovered until 1901, so it was not possible to match donor to recipient, with often catastrophic results. But Dr. Llewellyn Williams had another idea. A really rather strange one.

As a means which I believe will prove equally as powerful as
transfusion in arresting the vital spirit, I had recourse to ene-
mata of port wine, believing that this remedy possesses a three-
fold advantage. The stimulating and life-sustaining effects of
the wine are made manifest in the system generally; the appli-
cation of cold to the rectum excites the reflex action of the nerves
supplying the uterus; and the astringent property of port wine
may act beneficially by causing the open extremities of the ves-
sels themselves to contract.

Applying cold liquid to arrest bleeding was at least a rational thing to do: Crushed ice was often piled on top of the abdomen after childbirth if hemorrhage was difficult to arrest. But in other respects, the use of port in these circumstances has little to recommend it.

I commenced by administering about four ounces of port wine,
together with twenty drops of tincture of opium. It was interest-
ing to note the rapidity with which the stimulating effects of the
wine became manifest on the system.

After a brief improvement, the woman's pulse began to flag, so the doctor administered a second enema.

A more marked improvement was now manifest in the patient. She regained her consciousness; the pulse continued feebly perceptible at the wrist. In half an hour I had again recourse to the enema, with the most gratifying result; and, after ten hours' most anxious watching, I had the happiness of leaving my patient out of danger.

Whether Dr. Llewellyn Williams was in any way responsible for her improvement remains a moot point.

The quantity of wine consumed was rather more than an ordinary bottle.

Not the most pleasurable way of consuming a bottle of port, by any means.

There's a minor postscript to this unexpectedly happy ending: Six months after his article appeared in print, the *British Medical Journal* announced that Dr. Llewellyn Williams's wife had given birth to a son. Whether she was given rectal doses of port, brandy or any other stimulating alcoholic beverage is not recorded. For her sake, let's hope the good doctor left the delivery of his own child to one of his colleagues.

THE SNAKE-DUNG SALESMAN

In 1862, an Edinburgh-trained physician, Dr. John Hastings, published a slim volume about the treatment of tuberculosis and other diseases of the lung. It advocates the use of substances that much of the profession would regard as unorthodox, as he acknowledges in his preface:

It has been suggested that the peculiar character of these agents may possibly prove a bar to their employment for medicinal purposes.

Dr. Hastings then anticipates another likely objection—that the "medicine" he recommends is difficult to get hold of. Fear not: He can recommend some suppliers.

It may be useful to add that these new agents may chiefly be procured from the Zoological Gardens of London, Edinburgh, Leeds, Paris, and other large towns. They may also be obtained from the dealers in reptiles, two of whom—Jamrach and Rice*—reside in Ratcliffe-highway, whilst two or three others are to be found in Liverpool.

One might reasonably ask what sort of medicine can be purchased only at a zoo or pet shop. Dr. Hastings explains that he spent several years trying to find novel medicinal substances in nature, without success. Deciding that pharmacies were already "crowded with medicines derived from the vegetable and mineral world," he resolved to investigate possible miracle cures in the animal kingdom.

It would be foreign to my purpose to detail here the various animals I put in requisition in the course of this investigation, or the animal products I examined during a prolonged inquiry. It is enough to state that I found in the excreta of reptiles agents of great medicinal value in numerous diseases where much help was needed.

---

* Charles Jamrach was a German emigré who became the most successful trader of exotic animals in nineteenth-century England. His warehouse in Wapping, in London's docklands, contained an unlikely menagerie of lions, tigers, crocodiles, bears, zebras and numerous smaller fauna. Mr. Rice, a competitor who chose injudiciously to set up shop in the same street, has left barely any trace on the historical record.

Yes, Dr. Hastings's miracle cure was reptile excrement. His book is entitled

AN INQUIRY

INTO THE MEDICINAL VALUE

OF

THE EXCRETA OF REPTILES,

Which reptiles, you may be asking?

My earliest trials were made with the excreta of the boa constrictor, which I employed in the first instance dissolved simply in water. A gallon of water will not dissolve two grains, and yet, strange as the statement may appear, half a teaspoonful of this solution rubbed over the chest of a consumptive patient will give instantaneous relief to his breathing.

Not just the boa constrictor either. Dr. Hastings provides a list of the species whose droppings he has investigated: nine types of snake (including African cobras, Australian vipers and Indian river snakes), five varieties of lizard and two tortoises. After his eureka moment, the intrepid physician was eager to introduce the new medicinal agents into clinical practice, and so he started to prescribe reptile excrement for his patients. Since his specialty was tuberculosis, most of the people who came to see Dr. Hastings would have been scared and desperate. In the 1860s, there was no cure for TB; although it was not universally fatal, around half of those who contracted the disease would die, most of them within two years.

Dr. Hastings includes a number of case reports. The first concerns "Mr. P.," a twenty-eight-year-old musician who consulted him about a troublesome cough. Unexplained weight loss had eventually prompted the diagnosis of tuberculosis:

> *I prescribed the 200th part of a grain of the excreta of the monitor niloticus (warning lizard of the Nile) in a tablespoonful of water, to be taken three times a day, and directed an external application of the same solution to the diseased side. He was much better at the end of a week, and after a further week's treatment I lost sight of him in consequence of his believing himself cured.*

Another was "the Reverend Q.C.," who sought treatment after he started to cough up blood, the classic presentation of tuberculosis. He was treated with two different types of lizard poo:

> *I applied to the walls of the left chest a lotion composed of the excreta of the boa constrictor of the strength of the ninety-sixth part of a grain to half an ounce of water. Under this treatment his amendment made rapid progress, until the month of May, when I prescribed for him a solution of the excreta of the monitor niloticus (warning lizard of the Nile) of the strength of the 200th part of a grain in two teaspoonfuls of water three times a day, and directed him to use the same mixture externally.*

The clergyman's symptoms improved dramatically, and a few weeks later, he was able to walk eight or ten miles "with ease." But my favorite case is that of "Miss E.," described as a "public vocalist," which contains this magnificent paragraph:

This case is interesting, from the fact that I gave her the excreta of every serpent I have yet examined, and they all, without exception, after a few days' use, occasioned headache or sickness, with diarrhoea to such an extent that I was obliged to relinquish their use. From the excreta of the lizards she experienced no inconvenience. She is now taking the excreta of the chameleo vulgaris (common chameleon) with great advantage, and is better than she has been at any one period during the last three years.

It's all pretty ridiculous— a fact that the medical journals of the day did not fail to point out. A review in *The British Medical Journal* makes an excellent point about the nature of scientific evidence, suggesting that the "positive" results he recorded were nothing of the sort:

This doctor, unfortunately, gives his cases—his exempla to prove his thesis; and we must, indeed, announce them as such to be lamentable failures as supporters of his proposition. We verily believe, and we say it most conscientiously, that if Dr Hastings had rubbed in one-two-hundredth of a grain of cheese-parings, and had administered one-two-hundredth of a grain of chaff, and had treated his patients in other respects the same as he doubtless treated them, he would have obtained equally satisfactory results.

If *The British Medical Journal* was uncomplimentary, *The Lancet* was positively scathing. Its reviewer points out that twenty years earlier, Dr. John Hastings had published another book in which he claimed to be able to cure consumption—using naphtha.* And twelve years after *that*, he had decided that the cure for

---

* A flammable liquid hydrocarbon

consumption was "oxalic* and fluoric† acids"; oh yes, and "the bi-sulphuret of carbon."‡ Dr. Hastings had, in fact, discovered not one but *five* cures. The reviewer adds, with considerable sarcasm:

> *As regards that—to ordinary men—unmanageable malady, consumption, all our difficulties are now at an end. The public may fly to Dr Hastings this time with the fullest confidence that the great specific is in his grasp at last.*

But he saves the best till last:

> *What can the public be thinking about, we would ask, when it supports and patronizes such absurd doings? Will there still continue to be found persons ready to allow their sick friends to be washed with a lotion of serpents' dung?*

Dr. Hastings was so offended by this article that he attempted to sue the publisher of *The Lancet* for libel. The matter was heard before the Lord Chief Justice, Sir Alexander Cockburn, who dismissed the case, ruling:

> *It might be that he had discovered a remedy, and, if so, truth would prevail in the end; but it was not to be wondered at that the matter was treated rather sarcastically when the public were told that phthisis could be cured by the dung of snakes.*

Well said!

---

* Oxalic acid is present in many foods but toxic in high concentrations.
† Known today as hydrofluoric acid, and unspeakably bad for you in large doses. Even skin contact can be fatal.
‡ Carbon disulfide, a pleasant-smelling but highly toxic liquid

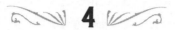

HORRIFYING
OPERATIONS

THE EIGHTEENTH-CENTURY NOVELIST Tobias Smollett was originally destined for a medical career. At the age of fifteen he was apprenticed to two Glasgow surgeons, and three years later volunteered for service in the Royal Navy. Before he could take up his position as second mate to a ship's surgeon, he first needed to pass an exam at the headquarters of the Company of Barber-Surgeons in London, where his inquisitors included William Chesclden, one of the great surgical innovators of the era. Smollett later satirized this occasion to comic effect in his novel *The Adventures of Roderick Random* (1748), in which one of the examiners asks the young Roderick what he would do if "during an engagement at sea, a man should be brought to you with his head shot off?" Random proves equal to this facetious challenge:

> *After some hesitation, I owned such a case had never come under my observation, neither did I remember to have seen any method of care proposed for such an accident, in any of the systems of surgery I had perused.*

In 1742, Smollett spent a year treating casualties onboard HMS *Chichester* during the war against Spain, and the squalor and suffering he witnessed onboard the man-of-war provided him with abundant raw material for *Roderick Random*. His descriptions of "pitiless surgery and amputation" (as Leigh Hunt described them to Shelley) are among the most vivid ever committed to paper.

The operations Smollett and his fictional alter ego performed in the heat of battle were primitive and mostly concerned with the treatment of wounds. Until the second half of the nineteenth century, when the advent of anesthetics and antisepsis vastly increased the scope of surgical intervention, the repertoire of procedures was small. The removal of cataracts was sometimes attempted in the eighteenth century, but major operations were largely limited to amputations and lithotomy, the removal of bladder stones.

But that's not the whole story. The early medical literature also contains numerous examples of surgeons attempting procedures that went far beyond the boundaries of what was considered orthodox or even possible. In 1817, thirty years before the discovery of anesthesia, the London surgeon Astley Cooper nearly succeeded in treating a large aneurysm by tying a ligature around the patient's abdominal aorta—an undertaking of such gravity that it was not attempted again for another century. In Cooper's age of so-called heroic surgery, many operations of comparable daring took place in front of a large audience, with patients who were horrifically conscious of all that was going on.

Some of these were misguided to the point of rashness, but others display a sophistication and skill not often associated with this early period in medical history. Desperation sometimes prompted surgeons to improvise a solution to a problem that had hitherto been thought insoluble. Necessity is famously the mother of invention, and in some of these cases, operations were performed by those who had never previously wielded a scalpel—and, on occasion, even by the patient on their own body.

But be in no doubt: Even when such procedures were successful, it was not a pleasant business. As the German Lorenz Heister, author of the most widely read surgical textbook of the eighteenth century, wrote:

> *Students in surgery should not only be furnished with strength of body, but constancy of mind also, that they may remain unmolested and unmoved by the stench, blood, pus, and nastiness that will naturally occur to them in their practice.*

And if that didn't put them off, nothing would.

THE CASE OF THE DRUNKEN DUTCHMAN'S GUTS

On August 28, 1641, the twenty-year-old English diarist John Evelyn visited the great university of Leiden in the Netherlands. He was unimpressed, declaring it "nothing extraordinary," but one building took his fancy:

> *Amongst all the rarities of this place, I was much pleased with a sight of their anatomy school, theatre, and repository adjoining, which is well furnished with natural curiosities. Amongst a great variety of other things, I was shown the knife newly taken out of a drunken Dutchman's guts, by an incision in his side, after it had slipped from his fingers into his stomach.*

This object evidently made quite an impression. More than twenty years later, Evelyn recorded the following exchange with the future King James II (James VII, if you're Scottish):

> *I had much discourse with the Duke of York, concerning strange cures he affirmed of a woman who swallowed a whole ear of barley, which worked out at her side. I told him of the KNIFE SWALLOWED and the pins.*

No wonder he remembered it: The case of the "drunken Dutchman's guts" was one of the most extraordinary medical events of the seventeenth century—an operation so daring that two hundred years later, in the era of anesthetics and aseptic surgery, it would still be regarded as a heroic achievement. In 1738, the professor of medicine at the University of Königsberg, Daniel Beckher, wrote a book about this case (in Latin) that became a bestseller across much of Europe. *De cultrivoro Prussiaco observatio* ("On the Knife-Eating Prussian") was translated into English as *A Miraculous Cure of the Prusian Swallow-Knife*, a copy of which eventually found its way into John Evelyn's library. Beckher's account goes into exhaustive detail, so here I'm relying on a more digestible (as it were) summary by Thomas Barnes written for *The Edinburgh Philosophical Journal* in 1824:

> *On the morning of the 29th of May 1635, Andrew Grünbeide, a young peasant, feeling sick at stomach from having committed some irregularity in his mode of living, endeavoured to excite vomiting by irritating the fauces with the handle of a knife . . .*

The fauces is the back of the throat. The original text makes clear that Herr Grünbeide had had far too much to drink the previous

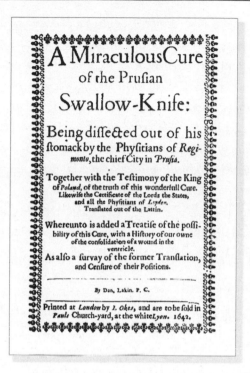

A MiraculousCure
of the Prusian
Swallow-Knife:

Being diffeƈted out of his
ſtomack by the Phyſitians of *Regimonto*, the chief City in *Pruſia*.

Together with the Teſtimony of the King
of *Poland*, of the truth of this wonderfull Cure.
Likewiſe the Certificate of the Lords the States,
and all the Phyſitians of *Leyden*.
Tranſlated out of the Lattin.

Whereunto is added a Treatiſe of the poſſibility of this Cure, with a Hiſtory of our owne
of the conſolidation of a wound in the
ventricle.
As alſo a ſurvay of the former Tranſlation,
and Cenſure of their Poſitions.

By Dan, Lakin. P. C.

Printed at *London* by *I. Okes*, and are to be ſold in
Pauls Church-yard, at the white *Lyon.* 1642.

night, and no doubt many students, past and present, will be familiar with this method of provoking vomiting. It is not recommended, particularly if you are stupid enough to use a knife.

> . . . *but the desired effect not being immediately produced, he thrust it further down, in consequence of which it escaped his hold, and gradually descended into the stomach. The knifeeater was terribly frightened at the time, and continued afterwards much depressed, yet was able to follow his accustomed employment without much inconvenience.*

It's difficult to imagine anybody in his position being anything other than "terribly frightened."

The wretched condition of this afflicted peasant excited much pity, and many physicians and surgeons of great learning and celebrity were consulted respecting him. At a meeting of the Faculty, held on the 25th of June, it was decided that the abdomen should be opened, an incision made into the stomach, and the knife extracted. Previous to the operation, the patient was to make use of a balsamic oil, called Spanish Balsam, which they supposed would alleviate the pains of the stomach, and facilitate the healing of the wound.

It was decided that the dreaded operation should take place on July 9. The original account (in its 1642 translation by Daniel Lakin) is vivid:

Of the very Incifion of the Ventricle, and extraction of the Knife.

There met therefore with the Dean of the faculty of physic, the most excellent physicians, honourable members of the same college, as also the students, masters of our Art, together with the most experienced surgeon and cutter of the stone, Mr Dan. Schwabius my gossip* and venerable friend now in Heaven.

It was quite a crowd of eminent medical men in the operating theater. When they were satisfied that everything was ready, they bowed their heads in prayer to invoke "divine assistance and benediction," and the operation could begin.

---

* An intimate acquaintance or friend

The rustic who with an undaunted courage waited the section* was bound to a wooden table, and the place being marked out with a coal, the incision was made towards the left side of the hypochondrium some two fingers' breadth under the short ribs.

In other words, the incision was made on the upper part of the abdomen, on the patient's left side.

First the skin and that fleshy pannicle (there was no fat seen) and then the subjected muscles, as also the peritoneum was cut and opened.

Pannicle is an archaic anatomical term meaning a layer of tissue. The peritoneum is the membrane lining the abdominal cavity. Thomas Barnes describes the climactic moment of this great endeavor:

The stomach subsided and slipped from the fingers, which prevented it from being immediately seized; but it was at length caught hold of with a curved needle, and drawn out of the wound. A small incision was then made into it upon the knife, which was then easily extracted . . .

In case you're wondering, yes, the patient was still awake. In 1635, he had little alternative, except perhaps passing out with the pain. But far from being in agonies, he was apparently the most enthusiastic spectator:

---

* I.e., awaited the operation

*... which was viewed by all that were standing by, and greatly
applauded both by them and the patient himself, who professed
that this was the very knife he some few days before had swallowed, but the wound itself when the knife was drawn forth
was quickly allayed.**

The English translation includes a frontispiece that shows the remarkable size of the knife and the incision from which it was removed.

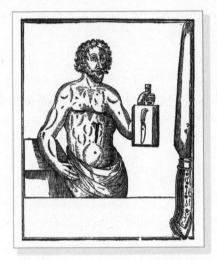

It would be reasonable to expect some pretty major complications
to follow an operation of such gravity, performed two hundred
years before the mechanisms of infection were understood. But this
patient enjoyed a near-miraculous recovery. The surgeon cleaned
the external wound and then stitched it with five sutures; "tepid
balsam" was poured on it before a dressing of clay, egg white and
alum was applied.

---

* Relieved, soothed

The following day, he was well enough to eat chicken broth, "boiled with bitter and astringent herbs," which doesn't sound like the sort of thing I'd want to eat straight after a stomach operation. After a week, his doctors declared him out of danger, and he was given rhubarb to aid his digestion.

The same treatment and dressing were continued until the 23rd of July, which was the 14th day after the operation, when the wound had healed, and nothing occurred afterwards worthy of notice. He was restored to the best of health, gradually returned to his ordinary diet and employment, and never afterwards complained of pains in his stomach.

And the knife? It was a fearsome object, described in a later article in the *Philosophical Transactions* as being six and a half inches long. The author of that article, Dr. Oliver, met a Scottish merchant living in Königsberg, who told him

that Andrew Grünbeide was his particular friend and acquaintance; that he saw his wound several times when his surgeons dressed him, and was godfather to one or two of his children after his recovery.

It's an amazing story, and a historic operation: Gastric surgery would remain a rare and risky undertaking until the twentieth century. For many years, the knife removed from the "drunken Dutchman's guts" was kept in a velvet bag in the king of Prussia's library—but the current whereabouts of this prize exhibit are, alas, unknown.

IF YOU CAN'T FIND A SURGEON . . .

. . . employ a butcher. That, at least, is the advice implied by this unusual eighteenth-century case from rural Ireland.

The village of Clogher in County Tyrone, Northern Ireland, is a bit of an oddity. Although it has never been much more than a hamlet, with barely five hundred residents even today, it also possesses a cathedral—one of the smallest settlements in the British Isles to do so. Between 1737 and 1743, the Dean of Clogher was John Copping, a keen amateur scientist who had been elected a Fellow of the Royal Society. In 1739, the society's journal, the *Philosophical Transactions*, published a pair of letters from the reverend gentleman. The first contains a story he'd been told by a young clergyman in the same diocese, who had briefly studied medicine and knew a little about it:

XVII. *Extraĉts of Two Letters from the Revd Dean* Copping, F. R. S. *to the* Prefident, *concerning the* Cæfarian *Operation performed by an ignorant Butcher; and concerning the extraordinary* Skeleton *mentioned in the foregoing Article.*

Sarah McKinna, who now lives at Brentram, two miles from the city of Clogher, in the county of Tyrone, was married at the age of sixteen years. Before her marriage she never had the appearance peculiar to women; but, in a month after her marriage, those appearances showed themselves properly.

A delicate way of saying that she had gone through puberty unusually late.

Ten months after her marriage, she found the symptoms of pregnancy, and bore a child at the expiration of the usual time. Ten months after, she was delivered of another; and each time had a speedy and easy delivery. Two months after her second lying-in, symptoms of pregnancy appeared again, and increased in proportion to the time; but at the end of nine months those symptoms began to dwindle, and in a little time she had no other reason for thinking she was with child, but an absolute stoppage of her catamenia.

She had stopped menstruating—and this symptom persisted for another six years, together with mysterious abdominal pains. And then a "swelling in her belly" led her to believe that she might once again be pregnant:

About seven months after this uncertain account, a boil, as she thought, appeared about an inch and a half higher than her navel. It was attended with very great pain. She sent for one Turlogh O'Neill, a butcher, who then did, and does now live with Capt. George Gledhames, about a mile from Clogher.

Why she sent for a butcher rather than a doctor is not explained. However, Mr. O'Neill duly arrived a few days later and found her "in an expiring condition":

By this time the impostumation* had broken, and an elbow of the child had forced itself through it, and appeared in view. At the request of herself and friends, he undertook to administer relief to her, and made so large an incision above and below the

---

* Abscess

navel, as enabled him, by fixing his fingers under the jaw of the
foetus, to extract it; in which operation he met not with the
least impediment.

Although it isn't spelled out, the implication here is that the fetus
had already died. That was bad enough; but far worse was to come.
Brace yourself.

He afterwards looked into her belly, and seeing something
black, he put in his hand, and extracted, by pieces, a perfect
skeleton of a child, and several pieces of black putrefied flesh.
After the operation, he swathed* her up; and in six weeks she
pursued her domestic business. She has been in good health
ever since this wonderful accident happened; only she has a
navel rupture, owing to the ignorance of the man in not apply-
ing a proper bandage.

The "navel rupture" was an umbilical hernia: The incision had
weakened the muscles of the abdominal wall, allowing a portion of
the intestines to bulge through them. It's a strange tale, and one
leaving many questions unanswered. Dean Copping was not one to
trust hearsay, and at the first opportunity, he went to visit the woman
and her husband to hear their own version of events. But his inter-
view with the couple did not provide complete enlightenment.

They are so ignorant that, with their bad language, I could not
make myself quite master of what they said; but, if they speak
true, there is something more surprising than the former ac-
count mentioned.

---

* Bandaged

These communication problems are immediately apparent in Copping's narrative, since its chronology is wildly at odds with the original version. The woman now told him that she had been married not for ten months, but for ten *years*, before first falling pregnant. She had gone into labor at the expected time, but the contractions ceased, the abdominal swelling disappeared and the midwife concluded that it was a "phantom" pregnancy—there had never been a fetus. Seven years later, Sarah McKinna conceived again, and prayed that this time she would deliver a healthy child without any alarms. But then, as she explained to Dean Copping, things went terribly wrong:

> *There was a swelling in her navel about the bigness of a goose-egg, which broke in a small orifice, of itself, and discharged a watery humour. She had a midwife, and three or four physicians, who gave her over, and left her as a dying woman. From this orifice started the elbow of a child, which hung some days by the skin, visible to abundance: at length she cut it off for her own relief.*

Imagine the sort of state you'd have to be in to do such a thing.

> *When O'Neill came she begged him to help her. The man was frightened, and went to sleep; but, when he got up, gave her a large draught of sack, and, I suppose, took one himself . . .*

Sack is a fortified white wine from Spain.* In the rural Ireland of the 1730s, a "large draught of sack" was the closest available thing

---

* The salary of the British poet laureate traditionally includes a butt (barrel) of sack, and even today, the incumbent receives part of her stipend in the form of six hundred bottles of sherry.

to an anesthetic and therefore the only viable way of mitigating the
pain. Having administered this dose, the butcher

> . . . *opened the place, and made such a hole as the man de-*
> *scribes to be as large as his hat.*

A vivid comparison, but not one you'd expect to read in a medical
paper.

> *He put in his hand, took hold of the second bone of the child,*
> *and, pulling it backward and forward to loosen it, in a little*
> *time extracted the child. After this, looking into the hole, and*
> *seeing something black, he put in his hand, and extracted other*
> *bones. Some bones still remained, which were extracted at dif-*
> *ferent times, it seems too in different ways; for some came by the*
> *navel, others from the womb the natural way.*

Dean Copping explains that these body parts continued to emerge
from the poor woman's body over a period of six months, from July
to Christmas.

> *She had great pain at each time. The former account says, she*
> *pursued her domestic business: she might be about the house, but*
> *she was fifteen months confined to the house. I have examined the*
> *rupture, and can put a finger a pretty way up into the body. Mr*
> *Dobbs, I hear, an eminent surgeon at Dublin, thinks there may*
> *be relief, and that the rupture may be much helped, and the guts*
> *reduced. I question whether he will think so, when he sees her.*

A laconic remark that implies she was in a very bad way. Dean Copping was a kindly man and was determined to do something to help.

I have collected about four pounds for her among the Gentlemen that visit my Lord Bishop, shall buy her some clothes, and send her to Dublin about ten days hence, to the infirmary. She was fond of going, but her ignorant priest, and some other ignorant neighbours, told her they would keep her till she dies.

Nothing like a bit of moral support, eh? Eventually, the woman and her husband were persuaded otherwise.

But, upon my answering those difficulties, she consents to go; her husband will carry her, and they are so thankful to me for entering so much into their condition that they now say she shall go to London, or wherever I please.

Sadly, there is no word as to what happened to the woman after her removal to Dublin; at this date, any further surgical intervention might easily have killed her. In rural areas, where surgeons were scarce and few could afford them, butchers must on occasion have been pressed into service instead—and being able to dismember a cow or pig would be a useful skill if you were suddenly asked to turn your hand to an amputation. But examples of butchers pursuing such extracurricular activities are thankfully rare in the medical literature.

THE SELF-INFLICTED LITHOTRIPSY

In 1961, a Russian scientist working at a remote base in the Antarctic fell seriously ill with an infected appendix. The weather was treacherous and there was no possibility of evacuation, so Leonid

Rogozov knew that the only option was for the team's medical officer to perform an appendectomy. Unfortunately, he *was* the medical officer, the one person within a thousand miles capable of doing
such a thing. So, aided by his colleagues and a little local anesthetic, Rogozov became the first surgeon to take out his own appendix.

Rogozov's auto-appendectomy is the best-known case of self-
surgery on record, but it's far from unique. A less bloody, but far
more prolonged, example took place in India in the eighteenth century. The patient (and surgeon) was Claude Martin, a French-born
colonel in the service of the British East India Company. As well as
enjoying a successful military career, he also worked as a cartogra-
pher, architect and administrator, becoming the richest European
in India. He also constructed—and flew—the first hot-air balloon in
India. A polymath and voracious reader, Martin bequeathed much
of his fortune to good causes, including the foundation of three
schools that still exist today.

In 1782, Martin developed the symptoms of a bladder stone,
and realized that unless he did something about it, he would have
to undergo surgery. This operation, known as lithotomy, is one of
the oldest in all the surgical canon. It would entail making an incision into the bladder and extracting the stone, a concretion of min-
erals from the urine. Ancient Indian and Greek doctors described
the procedure in some detail, and until 150 years ago, it was of
course conducted without anesthetic. It was dangerous and notoriously painful, and Colonel Martin was understandably reluctant to
put himself through the experience—so he decided to deal with the
problem himself. In 1799, he wrote a letter, subsequently published in a medical journal, explaining how he had taken matters
into his own hands:

Col. Martin, on destroying the Stone in the Bladder.

I have been so fortunate as to cure myself of the stone; which cure was, and must certainly appear very extraordinary to those who do not know how I accomplished it.

Colonel Martin's method involved inserting an instrument into his penis and up the urethra until it reached his bladder, and then filing the stone away, bit by bit. The file he used was one of his own making, consisting of a knitting needle set in a whalebone handle.

I began to file the stone in the bladder in April 1782, and as appears by a note I received from Doctor Rennet Murchison who was at this place as surgeon to the Resident, it soon made an impression upon the stone, and brought away many small pieces which are in my possession.

The plucky colonel sent one of these fragments to Dr. Murchison for his inspection. The doctor replied:

"Dear Martin, I have examined the stone with a good microscope; it seems to have a solid shell on the external part, but is internally of a loose texture. From this appearance I fancy your mechanical plan has had some effect; but, my dear friend, do not suffer yourself to be so sanguine in your hopes, as to use your file too often, for an inflammation in the bladder might now prove fatal; however, as the internal texture of the stone is loose, and as you have broken the hard surface on the outside, I have no doubt but you may get a great deal of it away, by the cautious use of your instrument."

What had he started? Dr. Murchison strongly disapproved of Colonel Martin's plan; but the intrepid Frenchman was not to be deterred.

This good man, Doctor Murchison, endeavoured to dissuade me from going on, but as I found daily the good effect of my filing, and never suffered particular pain in doing it, I persevered till the middle of October of the same year, and I think I filed, on an average, at the rate of at least three times in the twenty-four hours.

Yes, that's right: Three times a day he voluntarily inserted a knitting needle up his own urethra and had a good scrape. If that doesn't make you wince, I don't know what would.

I was at first puzzled how to bring the stone to the neck of the bladder, but I contrived to inject warm water into the bladder, which, endeavouring to discharge, it protruded the stone to its neck; I then introduced my file between the flesh and the stone, keeping my body inclined against a wall all the time, till by a bad stroke I pushed the stone from the neck of the bladder.

Was this *really* better than undergoing a painful ten-minute operation?

Fear of inflammation I had none; for it once happened that a spasm of the whole urethra fixed my file so firmly that I could not move it. This spasm lasted about ten minutes, and, when relaxed, a great deal of blood came away, and also many small pieces of the stone. In a couple of days, I could renew my filing without any pain, which convinced me that there was no fear

*of inflammation, and such spasms happened often without
any bad consequence.*

So that's all right, then.

*I am convinced that all persons may cure themselves, as it re-
quires very little address. I do not think it possible for another
to operate, as none but the patient can know where it pains
him, and he will naturally know, when and how he can introduce the file, as he cannot do it to any purpose, but when the
stone is at or near the neck of the bladder. The file being so very
small (not thicker than a straw), is easily introduced between
the fleshy part and the stone, and the motion in filing does not
extend beyond the length of about half an inch.*

Colonel Martin evidently had great confidence in the procedure he
had invented, but I must say I'm a long way from being convinced.
He then explains that he had previously been given conventional
treatments (mainly emetics and laxatives) by Dr. Murchison, which
had only made him sicker. The complaint was so painful that the
colonel had had to give up eating anything containing salt or spices.

*My food was nothing else but boiled or roasted meat, and water
for my drink, taking care to keep my body open by gentle laxatives. But, as soon as the urine became clear, my stomach began to be better, and I grew more easy, and more regular in
filing the stone, which I did very often in the day and night,
sometimes ten or twelve times in the day, and passed almost
every day small pieces, till the whole came away: and, as I said
above, I have been very well since; never had any pain, or return of stone or gravel till very lately.*

The article concludes with a letter from Warren Hastings, a friend of Martin's and the most senior British administrator in India during this period (he was famously accused of corruption, put on trial and acquitted by Parliament). Hastings writes:

> *I return you many thanks for the perusal of Colonel Martin's curious letter; for curious and interesting it is, even to me, who well remember all the particulars of his case, as he has detailed it to you, and even the language in which he has delivered them. I mentioned the fact once to Mr Pott, who evidently shewed, by his looks and silence, that he did not believe it.*

Percivall Pott was one of the leading surgeons of the day, best known for noticing that chimney sweeps were particularly prone to scrotal carcinoma—the first occupational cancer ever identified. His disbelief is understandable, since Colonel Martin was breaking new surgical ground. Until the 1820s, the only effective treatment for a patient with bladder stones was lithotomy, which involved extracting the object through an incision, with all the concomitant risks. But in the first half of the nineteenth century, several experts developed methods of drilling, grinding or crushing stones using instruments inserted through the urethra, avoiding open surgery entirely. The first such operation, which became known as lithotripsy, was performed in 1824 by the French surgeon Jean Civiale. Colonel Martin anticipated this breakthrough by forty years—and, not content with being the pioneering surgeon, he also volunteered to be his own first patient. And why not?

A HIGH PAIN THRESHOLD

In the late 1870s, an elderly retired surgeon from Birmingham, Dickinson Webster Crompton, was persuaded to write a short memoir. The friend who suggested it, a lecturer at Guy's Hospital in London, had been fascinated by his older colleague's tales about the operating theater of half a century earlier and thought they should be preserved for posterity. Crompton studied in London, Bonn and Paris, where his teachers had included Guillaume Dupuytren, the doyen of French surgery. But after completing his training, he returned to Birmingham, the city of his birth, where he pursued a happy and successful career until his retirement. By the age of seventy-three, he was almost completely blind, telling his friend that

> *I am now getting cataracts in my eyes, and at the present moment do not see what my hand writes, but hope it forms the words my mind would dictate.*

In 1878, Crompton's "Reminiscences of Provincial Surgery" was published in *Guy's Hospital Reports*, the institution's house journal. It provides a vivid account of early-nineteenth-century medical life in the West Midlands.

REMINISCENCES OF PROVINCIAL SURGERY

UNDER

SOMEWHAT EXCEPTIONAL CIRCUMSTANCES.

———

BY "AN OLD GUY'S MAN."
DICKINSON CROMPTON, F.R.C.S., Birmingham.

Crompton was in his forties when chloroform and ether first made their appearance, and he records the novelty of operating on a patient who was unconscious and unable to feel pain. But in the early part of his career, no such luxuries existed, and most of the operations he narrates took place without the benefit of anesthetics. They include this startling case of a double leg amputation:

A man of intemperate habits, living at Tamworth, lay drunk during a frosty night with his feet in a puddle by the railway. His feet were frozen in the morning, and eventually sloughed off, the integument closing in a conical form, leaving the extremities of the tibia and fibula exposed and carious.

Carious means "decaying." There's something shockingly casual about the statement that "his feet . . . eventually sloughed off," as if it were a snake losing its skin.

I heard of the case, and recommended him to be brought to the Birmingham General Hospital. When I saw the case I was astonished at the wonderful effort of nature towards cure. If the bones could have borne ferules like a walking-stick, being placed on them, the man would have been able to walk as well or better than on wooden legs.

Now, that would have been a sight worth seeing.

However, that could not be, so the man and I agreed that I should amputate the legs at the usual place, leaving him good stumps and the knees, whereupon to place the common wooden leg. I removed one first, the man sitting on the table and holding the thigh himself and looking on. Not a sound escaped him, but, when done, he said, "By gam! It is sharp."

By which, it seems, he was describing the keenness of the saw blade rather than the pain.

After three weeks' time I removed the other leg in the same manner, except that the man thought the saw did not cut well.

A real connoisseur!

When he was nearly ready to leave his bed he again took me into his consultation as to the inconvenience of the length of the common wooden leg, and asked to have them made only nine inches long, as then, "when he had grog aboard," he should not have so far to fall!

A very practical sentiment.

He lived years after, and was well known as a tramp, I think.

Dickinson Crompton follows that anecdote with one about a patient who showed even more impressive stoicism:

> *Some years ago I was called in the night to go to Meriden to an accident, prepared to amputate. I found a poor labourer lying on his cottage bed, his left arm hanging over the edge of the bed, dropping blood into a chamber-pot. A tourniquet was tightly placed just below the shoulder-joint; the arm was black, as if already mortified. I heard that the man's arm had been caught in the cog-wheel of one of the agricultural machines, and was drawn in up to the shoulder.*

In the circumstances, there was no alternative but to amputate the mangled limb, as close to the shoulder joint as possible.

> *There was no room for a tourniquet; and I requested Mr Clark, the surgeon of the village, to press upon the artery against the head of the bone.*

The artery in question is the axillary, a major vessel that supplies the arm. Usual practice during amputation was to use a tourniquet to prevent major bleeding; on this occasion, there was no room for one, so instead, they were forced to compress the artery with a finger. Once the limb had been cut off, it would be permanently tied shut.

> *There was a boy in the room, an apprentice, I was told, but he declined to come near the patient to hold out the arm. I was therefore obliged to hold the artery against the head of the bone with my left hand, while Mr Clark held the arm out at full length by the hand; but he told me he always "fainted at the sight of blood", so turning his face and body away as far as*

possible, he held on till I had made my incision and sawn through the bone as high as I could.

You'd think that fainting at the sight of blood might be a significant handicap to being an early-nineteenth-century surgeon, but apparently not.

There was only a cottage candle in the room, and therefore I asked Mr Clark to hold it, so that I could look for the arteries, but he had had enough. The poor patient was sitting on a chair making no complaint; in fact I think there could not have been much pain felt, from the appearance of the parts, so he himself said, "Sir, if you will give me the candle, I think I can hold it"; this he did, bringing his right hand round with the candle in it, so that I had a good view of the face of the stump.

Holding a candle with one arm, so that a surgeon can see well enough to finish amputating the other, takes some courage.

The man recovered, but I heard he died of phthisis* six months afterwards; indeed, he was phthisical at the time of the operation.

Rotten luck.

A WINDOW IN HIS CHEST

Occasionally, a surgeon performs a feat so impressive that the operation becomes permanently associated with their name. In 1817,

---

* Tuberculosis

the English surgeon Sir Astley Cooper astonished his colleagues by tying a ligature around a patient's abdominal aorta, the largest blood vessel in the abdomen. His patient (who was being treated for a large aneurysm in his groin) died, but the attempt was so widely admired for its audacity that for many years afterward, it was referred to simply as Sir Astley Cooper's operation.

The year after this celebrated failure, medics across Europe thrilled to news of another heroic surgical intervention. Accounts were printed in all the major journals, headlined "Richerand's Operation." The hero this time was Baron Anthelme Balthasar Richerand, a prominent Parisian surgeon ennobled by Louis XVIII for his tireless work treating casualties during the Napoleonic Wars. Richerand was an admirer of Sir Astley Cooper, even to a fault: He later fell out of favor in France after daring to suggest that the surgeons of his own country were inferior to those of England. His eponymous operation was every bit as astonishing as Sir Astley's— not to mention the fact that his patient actually survived. This is how *The Medico-Chirurgical Journal* described his triumph:

Case of Excision of a Portion of the Ribs, and also of the Pleura.
By CHEVALIER RICHERAND,
Professor of the Faculty of Medicine, and Chief Surgeon to the Hospital of Saint Louis.

M. Michelleau, a health officer of Nemours, was affected during three years with a cancerous tumour over the region of the heart, which was extirpated in the month of January, 1818; but a bleeding fungus was frequently reproduced, notwithstanding the application of cauteries and caustics.

Not a fungus as we'd understand it today, but in the old medical sense of an unwanted growth. The measures applied in the first attempts to eliminate the recurrence of the tumor were cautery (searing with a hot implement) and caustics (corrosive chemicals used to burn away the affected flesh).

> *He now came to Paris and M. Richerand found an enormous fungus rising from the wound, and discharging a reddish and horribly foetid sanies.* Yet the patient did not suffer much pain.*

M. Michelleau had a chronic cough but was otherwise in fairly robust health. An operation would be a daunting challenge, but the patient seemed strong enough to withstand it.

> *It was therefore determined to remove a portion of rib or ribs, if necessary, as the seat of disease was considered to be there. Professor Dupuytren, and other surgeons of distinction, were present, and assisted at this formidable operation.*

Baron Guillaume Dupuytren was the leading surgeon in Paris, and celebrated throughout Europe. He is principally remembered today for having given his name to Dupuytren's contracture, a condition in which the proliferation of benign tumors in the connective tissues of the hand make the fingers contract toward the palm, giving them a clawlike appearance. A few years later, the two baron-surgeons, Dupuytren and Richerand, would fall out spectacularly over Richerand's insult to the French surgical profession; but for now, at least, they were friendly collaborators. The patient was

---

* A thin, blood-tinged liquid discharged from ulcers or infected wounds

secured to the table to ensure that his movements would not disturb the operators. There was, after all, no anesthesia in 1818.

> *I commenced (says M. Richerand) by enlarging the wound through the medium of a crucial* incision, and discovered the sixth rib enlarged and red for four inches in length. With a bistoury I separated the attachments of the intercostal muscles, above and below, through this space, and then with a small Hey's saw I cut through the rib in two places and removed the diseased portion, carefully detaching, by means of a spatula, the costal pleura from the internal face of the rib.*

This was difficult and sophisticated surgery. Richerand realized that he needed to remove a section of cancerous rib, which entailed dissecting away the muscles and other structures attached to it, such as the pleura, the protective membrane covering the lungs. The instrument he used to saw through the bone, invented a few years earlier by the English surgeon William Hey, had a long handle and a blade only a few inches long. It was designed for opening the skull, but its small cutting edge made it ideal for this particular task.

> *The seventh rib was now found to be diseased, to an equal extent, and was removed in a similar manner, but with much more difficulty, and not without penetrating the cavity of the chest by a slight rent in the pleura. This membrane itself was now discovered to be in a thickened, diseased state; and, in short, to be the tissue whence the fungous vegetation sprang. It*

---

* In the shape of a cross

was diseased eight square inches in extent! To leave this behind was to leave the operation unfinished, and therefore the whole of it was removed by the scissors.

The operation now entered a still more dangerous phase. Puncturing the pleura allows air into the cavity around the lungs; this increase in pressure can cause one or both lungs to collapse, a condition known as pneumothorax. This is less of a threat in the modern operating room because chest surgery is undertaken with mechanical ventilation: The lungs are inflated and deflated automatically via a tube passed down the windpipe. M. Richerand had no such modern luxuries: If both his patient's lungs collapsed, there was little chance he would survive.

Not a drop of blood was lost. At this moment the air rushed in, the left lung collapsed, and, with the heart enveloped in its pericardium, pressed and presented itself at the wound.

A dramatic spectacle. The (conscious) patient's beating heart was now visible through the operative incision, while a collapsed lung posed an immediate threat to his life.

The wound was instantly covered with adhesive pluster to prevent suffocation. The anxiety and difficulty of breathing were now extreme, and continued so for twelve hours after the operation. The patient passed the night erect, and without sleep.

This is hardly surprising. Even if he had been comfortable enough to sleep, sheer terror would surely have prevented him from doing so.

Towards the morning sinapisms* were applied to the soles of the feet, and insides of the thighs, rendering the breathing easier. From this moment the pulse rose and the strength increased. The patient was kept on liquids. Three days passed thus. The fever was moderate, but the oppression of the breath was sufficient to prevent sleep. Ninety-six hours after the operation, we removed the dressings. The pericardium and lung had contracted adhesions round the circumference of the wound, which now formed a kind of window, through which we distinctly saw the action of the heart through its transparent covering.

That would be a great icebreaker at parties, wouldn't it? Imagine being introduced to a fellow guest whose heart was visible through his chest.

Fortunately, the adhesion of the heart to the lung was not complete, and left a sufficient passage for a copious serous discharge which issued from the wound for ten or twelve days, in the quantity of half a pint a day. On the 13th day this discharge ceased; and by the 18th day, the adhesion between the pericardium and lung was complete, and no air entered from without after that period. The patient could now lie down and sleep; his appetite and strength returned; the wound healed, and he perfectly recovered.

Adhesion is being used here in a technical sense: After surgery, the formation of scar tissue can cause adjacent structures to stick together. In this case, it had a beneficial effect, the adhesion between

---

* Plasters smeared with mustard paste, intended to cause the sensation of burning. According to a doctrine fashionable at the time and known as counter-irritation, a malady in one part of the body could be cured by creating an artificial "irritation" in another.

the lung and the sac around the heart forming an airtight seal that allowed the patient to breathe normally once again.

This was an astonishing outcome, but it's not quite the end of the story. In a more detailed account of the operation and its aftermath, subsequently translated in *The Edinburgh Medical and Surgical Journal*, M. Richerand gives this sequel:

> *The patient, who for some days had been making trial of his strength in a garden belonging to the house in which he lived, could not resist the desire of traversing in a carriage the streets of the capital. Not being fatigued by an excursion of five hours, during which he visited l'Ecole de Medicine, and caused to be shown him the portions of the ribs and pleura, which are deposited in the Museum of that establishment...*

If a large portion of my rib cage had been cut out without anesthetic, and was now on display at a medical museum, I'm fairly sure I'd go and have a look at it.

> *... there was nothing to prevent his returning home, where he arrived safely on the twenty-seventh day after the operation, having provided himself with a piece of boiled leather to cover the cicatrix* when healed.*

An understandable precaution. One final detail of this case intrigued M. Richerand. By the early nineteenth century, it was generally accepted that the surface of the heart had no pain receptors—that one could, therefore, touch the organ without discomfort. Chances to

---

* Scar

have a feel of a living human heart being few and far between, Richerand made sure to satisfy himself on this point.

I did not let slip the opportunity here offered of again proving the perfect insensibility of the heart and pericardium.

An oddity that should not be allowed to overshadow a titanic surgical achievement. As the anonymous correspondent in *The Edinburgh Medical and Surgical Journal* points out, the entire operation was fraught with difficulty. Richerand's account of sawing through and removing the patient's ribs makes no mention of the fact that there are many important blood vessels in the area—some of them actually running along grooves in the underside of the bones. To remove sections of rib, he had to dissect these free and tie them to prevent catastrophic blood loss. And he achieved this miracle with a patient who was fully conscious. Though this report doesn't mention it, the patient was himself a surgeon; I'd like to think this helped him get through his ordeal, but somehow I doubt it.

THE SAD CASE OF HOO LOO

One of the most striking recent developments in health care has been the rapid expansion of medical tourism. It's estimated that every year as many as 15 million people now travel abroad in order to seek treatment. Those who live in countries where private health care is the norm may be looking for a cheaper option; others go in search of drugs or surgery not available closer to home. You might assume that the possibility of traveling halfway across the world for a lifesaving operation only arose in the era of the jet airliner, but as long ago as 1831, a young man from China did exactly that.

His name was Hoo Loo, and his case caused a sensation. Some months earlier, he had walked from his village to the Macao Ophthalmic Hospital, the first Western hospital built in China for the benefit of the Chinese. He must have presented quite a sight, because his scrotum had swollen to grotesque proportions, apparently the result of a condition known as elephantiasis.* The hospital's founder and surgeon, Dr. Thomas Richardson Colledge, believed that the unnatural growth could be removed, but it was not a job that he was prepared to undertake. So he paid for Hoo Loo's passage to London, and gave him a letter of introduction to his old mentor at Guy's Hospital, Sir Astley Cooper.

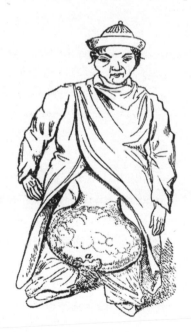

Contemporary engraving of Hoo Loo shortly before operation

---

* Also known as lymphatic filariasis, and caused by the parasitic roundworm *Wuchereria bancrofti*. But this diagnosis is uncertain; it may simply have been an enormous tumor.

His arrival prompted newspaper headlines, and the Chinese patient with the hideous deformity even inspired a political cartoon laboriously satirizing the attempts of the prime minister, Lord Grey, to pass his Reform Act. But the medics wasted no time in getting him treated, as *The Lancet* reported in April 1831:

> ## GUY'S HOSPITAL.
> ——
> **REMOVAL OF A TUMOUR FIFTY-SIX POUNDS IN WEIGHT, EXTENDING FROM BENEATH THE UMBILICUS TO THE ANTERIOR BORDER OF THE ANUS.**

Hoo Loo, a Chinese labourer, was admitted into Luke's ward, Guy's Hospital, in the third week of March last, with an extraordinary tumour depending from the lower part of the abdomen, and of a nature and extent hitherto unseen in this country.

Hoo Loo's tumor was simply enormous. It had started to appear ten years earlier, when he was twenty-two, as a small growth on the foreskin. By the time of the operation, it was four feet in circumference, hanging from the abdomen between the navel and the anus—almost entirely engulfing his genitals. The tumor was later found to weigh fifty-six pounds, and so disturbed his balance that Hoo Loo had to throw his shoulders backward while walking to compensate.

We have heard that on his voyage here the change of air had such an effect on his constitution, as to occasion a material increase in the tumour. Since his arrival his appetite, health, and spirits, were extremely good. While in the hospital there appeared nothing to induce the surgeon to order him any med-icine. His diet consisted principally of boiled rice, and no re-straint was placed on his appetite, which was very great. He was generally considered to have improved in health while in the hospital, though it was difficult to form a decided estimate on this point. He all along contemplated the operation with satisfaction.

Poignantly, Hoo Loo told one well-wisher that he intended to have the operation so that "he might prove a comfort to his aged mother, instead of being a burden to her." The procedure was scheduled for a Tuesday, but when the hospital authorities realized that a large crowd of spectators was likely to attend, they moved it to a Satur-day in the hope that this would deter them:

Notwithstanding this precaution, however, an assemblage unprecedented in numbers on such an occasion presented them-selves for admission at the operating theatre, which was in-stantly filled in every part, although none but pupils, and of those only such as could at the moment present their "hospital tickets", were admitted.

"Hospital tickets" were issued to medical students and entitled them to watch operations for educational benefit.

Hundreds of gentlemen were consequently excluded, and it be-came obvious to the officers of the hospital that some other room must be selected. Accordingly Sir Astley Cooper entered, and, addressing the pupils, said that in consequence of the crowd, the patient being in a state which would admit of the removal, the operation would take place in the great anatomical theatre. A tremendous rush to that theatre accordingly took place, where accommodation was afforded to 680 persons, and where preparations were immediately made for the patient.

A microbiologist's nightmare—hundreds of people, all exhaling their germs in close proximity to an open wound. It was not until the 1860s that surgeons would pay any attention to maintaining sterile conditions in the operating theater. Hoo Loo entered the room and was secured on the table:

A short consultation now took place between Sir Astley Cooper, Mr Key, and Mr Callaway, during which it was finally agreed, that if it were found possible, the genital organs should be preserved. The face of the patient was then covered, and Mr Key, taking his station in front of the tumour, commenced the operation.

Charles Aston Key, the surgeon who took the lead on this occasion, was a former pupil of Sir Astley Cooper and was married to his niece. A tall man with an aristocratic air, he was also known for his short temper. This operation would try his patience to the limit. In brief, the plan was to excise the tumor while liberating the penis and testicles from their fleshy prison. Key began the procedure by making three large incisions, forming flaps of muscle and skin that would eventually be used to cover the gaping hole left when the growth had been removed. This must have been agonizing, since there was no anesthetic.

The operator then proceeded to lay bare the two [spermatic] cords and the penis, a step in the operation which was performed with very great neatness. Sufficient time had now elapsed for the depressing effects of the operation to exhibit themselves, while the penis and testicles had yet to be dissected out. The determination to attempt this arose from its having been ascertained that the sexual inclinations of the man were unimpaired, seminal emissions being occasionally experienced. The delay, however, which so intricate a portion of the operation would have occasioned, now induced Sir Astley Cooper to propose that the genital organs should be sacrificed, and the suggestion was promptly acceded to.

This may seem a brutal decision, but the procedure was a battle against the clock. Their patient was enduring unimaginable pain, and if they took too long, he could die from hemorrhage or shock. Taking this grim shortcut allowed them to get on with the main business of dissecting out the tumor, a painstaking process that entailed tying off a number of blood vessels.

But a period of time elapsed before the conclusion of the operation which must have far exceeded the anticipations even of the most fearful, and by the time the tumour was entirely separated and the exposed parts were closed over, an hour and forty-four minutes had passed. This tremendous protraction was chiefly occasioned by the intervals which were from time to time allowed the patient for recovery from the fits of exhaustion which supervened.

Understandably. In an age when surgeons prided themselves on being able to amputate a limb in a couple of minutes, an operation lasting an hour and three-quarters was something quite out of the ordinary. Hoo Loo fainted several times, and in the latter stages, he was almost entirely unconscious. He had lost a fair amount of blood, although those present estimated that it was barely more than a pint.

> *Immediately after the removal of the tumour, another fit of syncope*—if syncope could be said to be at all incomplete for the last half hour—came on, from which the poor fellow did not for a moment rally. No remedies that were directed to overcome this state of collapse had the slightest effect; warmth and friction of the extremities, warmth to the scrobiculis cordis,† the injection of brandy and water into the stomach, and, ultimately, from the suspicion that the loss of blood had been too great, transfusion to the amount of six ounces, taken from the arm of a student—one amongst several who offered to afford blood—were amongst the means resorted to.*

This really was a last throw of the dice. Blood transfusion had been employed successfully in humans only a few times before; the physician responsible for these attempts, James Blundell, was also on the staff at Guy's. The operation often failed because the blood of donor and recipient were incompatible.

> *The heart's action gradually and perceptibly sunk. The patient did breathe after the operation, but that is as much as can be said. Artificial respiration was subsequently, but vainly attempted.*

---

* Unconsciousness
† Pit of the stomach

The unnamed author of this report adds a tribute to the tragic but courageous patient:

> *The fortitude with which this great operation was approached, and throughout undergone, by Hoo Loo, was, if not unexampled, at all events never exceeded in the annals of surgery. A groan now and then escaped him, and now and then a slight exclamation, and we thought we could trace in his tones a plaintive acknowledgment of the hopelessness of his case. Expressions of regret, too, that he had not rather borne with his affliction than suffered the operation, seemed softly but rapidly to vibrate from his lips as he closed his eyes, firmly set his teeth, and resignedly strung every nerve in obedience to the determination with which he had first submitted to the knife.*

Though admiring Aston Key's skill, a *Lancet* editorial was highly critical of the time he took to perform the operation, and the "obnoxious atmosphere" caused by the presence of more than six hundred spectators in the room. But that was as nothing to the response of a surgeon who wrote to the journal the following week. "Modern surgery is a vampire which feasts upon human blood,"* wrote Mr. Simpson, launching into a ferocious attack upon his colleagues:

> *I trust that nature was more merciful than man, and from the extremity of his sufferings formed a veil of oblivion, which rendered this unfortunate being at least partially insensible to his agonies. I think that this operation could neither advance the science of surgery, nor be otherwise beneficial to the human*

---

* Quoting John Armstrong, a maverick antiestablishment physician of the early nineteenth century

*race; that it was neither sanctioned by reason, nor warranted
by experience.*

As Simpson pointed out, the patient's life had not been in imminent danger; the decision to operate may have had more to do with
surgical hubris than clinical need. The death of Hoo Loo prompted
a period of soul-searching among the English medical profession—
and hastened the end of the "heroic" era of surgery, when interven-
tions were sometimes valued more highly for their dramatic impact
than for their effect on the patient. Too late, alas, for the unfortunate Chinese peasant who had traveled thousands of miles in the
forlorn hope of a cure.

ALL AT SEA

When I first came across this stirring tale of improvised surgery at
sea, I wasn't at all sure that it could be true. It appeared in 1853 in
a minor journal called *The Scalpel*, which was published in New
York between 1849 and 1864. The magazine was edited, and
mostly written, by the indefatigable Dr. Edward H. Dixon, a highly
regarded expert on sexually transmitted diseases and an outspo-
ken opponent of masturbation—a practice that, according to many
doctors of the era, led to illness and even death.

The Scalpel was unlike other medical journals in that it was
aimed at lay readers as well as professionals. Its articles were con-
versational, avoided unnecessary jargon and were often satirical in
intent. At first glance, this story looks like one of Dixon's humorous
jeux d'esprit, but much of the detail is corroborated by contemporary newspaper reports and even shipping records.

Extraordinary Operation on the Subclavian Vein, by the Mate of a Vessel ; Recovery.

Edward T. Hinckley, of Wareham, Mass., then mate of the bark Andrews, commanded by James L. Nye, of Sandwich, Mass., sailed some two years and a half since (we find the date omitted in our minutes) from New Bedford, Mass., on a whaling voyage.

New Bedford was probably the busiest whaling port in the world at the time, with eighty-seven ships setting off on expeditions in 1850 alone. One of them, the *Ann Alexander*, would become famous the following year when she was rammed and sunk by a sperm whale— a real-life Moby Dick!* Very few ships are known to have been sunk by whales, but on its voyage, the *Andrews*—which weighed anchor just two days after the *Ann Alexander*—would also have an unfortunate encounter with one. During an eventful voyage, it was the crew, however, who provided the early excitement:

When off the Galapagos Islands, one of the hands, who had shown a mutinous disposition, attacked Captain Nye with some violence, in consequence of a reproof given him for disobedience. In the scuffle which ensued, a wound was inflicted with a knife, commencing at the angle of the jaw, and dividing the skin and superficial tissues of the left side of the neck, down to

---

* The parallel is not entirely fanciful: Melville's masterpiece was already written but not yet published, and in a contemporary letter, the author commented that the sinking was "really & truly a surprising coincidence . . . I wonder if my evil art has raised this monster."

*the middle of the clavicle, under which the point of the knife
went.*

An ugly-sounding wound. The knife opened up a gash down the
side of the captain's neck, from the hinge of his jaw to the col-
larbone.

*It was done in broad day, in presence of the greater part of the
crew; and Mr. Hinckley, the mate, being so near that he was at
that moment rushing to the captain's assistance. Instantly seizing the villain, and handing him over to the crew, the knife either fell or was drawn by someone present, and a frightful gush
of dark blood welled up from the wound, as the captain fell
upon the deck.*

The "dark blood" was a sign that a vein, rather than an artery, had
been injured—still serious, but less immediately life-threatening.

*Mr. Hinckley immediately thrust his fingers into the wound,
and endeavored to catch the bleeding vessel; with the thumb
against the clavicle, as a point of action, and gripping, as he
expressed it to me, "all between," he found the bleeding nearly
cease. Such had been the violence of the haemorrhage, a space
on the deck fully as large as a barrel head being covered with
blood in a few seconds, that it was evident from that and the
consequent faintness that the captain would instantly die,
should he remove his fingers from the bleeding vessel.*

An alarming position to be in. His finger was now holding back a
crimson tide, like a bloodier version of the little Dutch boy and the
dyke. He paused for a moment to work out what to do.

The bleeding had stopped for now, but he needed to find a way of removing his digits without the hemorrhage recurring:

"I found my fingers passed under something running in the same course with the bone; this I slowly endeavored to draw up out of the wound, so as to see if it was not the blood vessel. Finding it give a little, I slowly pulled it up with one finger; when I was pulling it up, the captain groaned terribly, but I went on, because I knew I could do nothing else. As soon as I could see it, I washed away the blood, and was astonished and very glad to see there were two vessels, as I supposed them to be, one behind the other: the cut was in the front one."

This clear description makes it possible to identify the blood vessels as the subclavian vein and its associated artery. Both lie just underneath the clavicle, the vein in front of the artery. The subclavian artery is one of the major branches of the aorta: If it, rather than the vein, had been punctured, the captain would probably have bled to death within a few minutes. What would you do in such desperate circumstances? I'd probably yell for help, loudly. But Mr. Hinckley was made of sterner stuff.

"As I had often sewed up cuts in the flesh, and knew nothing about tying blood vessels, and supposed that was only done when they were cut in two, as in amputated limbs, I concluded to try my hand at sewing it up; so I took five little stitches; they were very near together, for the wound was certainly not half an inch wide, if so much."

Mr. Hinckley was evidently skillful with a needle and thread, because this sounds ferociously difficult. Remember, he was standing

on the deck of a moving ship, having only just averted a mutiny—
hardly the easiest circumstances for fine suture work.

*On inquiry of Mr. Hinckley, if he cut off the thread each time
and threaded the needle again, he said Yes; but "I only cut off
one end, and left the other hanging out." This he had learned
from a little book, prepared for the use of sea captains and
others, when no surgeon was on board.*

It sounds as if Mr. Hinckley was a quick learner. He used an "inter-
rupted" suture technique: Each stitch was separate from its neigh-
bor. It was standard practice at the time to leave the threads
dangling out through the wound—this allowed the surgeon to remove or tighten them as necessary.

*Mr. H. continued: "I twisted the ends together loosely, so as to
make one large one, and let it hang out of the wound over the
bone; then I closed all up with stitches and plasters. On the
fourteenth day I found the strings loose in the wound, from
which matter had freely come: it healed up like any other cut."*

And that was that: a complete recovery. But having cheated death
once, the captain was less fortunate the next time.

*Poor Captain Nye finally met a sad fate; he was drowned on the
destruction of his boat by an enraged whale.*

It's difficult to establish precisely what happened. Captain Nye and
two of his men were indeed killed by a whale on December 29,
1852, but the vessel returned to port on May 3 the following year,
minus a captain but carrying 909 barrels of sperm oil. The

Andrews then apparently went back to sea and was "lost on the Galapagos" sometime later that year. Of Mr. Hinckley's subsequent fate nothing is known, although I suspect he left the ship in May 1853, since his account of the operation in *The Scalpel* appeared some months later.

The article concludes in grandiose manner:

> *We may be mistaken in our views of its importance, but we think that in the estimation of our professional readers we have placed upon record one of the most extraordinary circumstances in the whole history of Surgery.*

Dr. Dixon has a point. Suturing veins and arteries was a notoriously difficult thing to do, and it was not until the beginning of the twentieth century that a surgeon succeeded in joining the two ends of a completely severed vessel. A specialist at any of the great hospitals of London, New York or Paris would have been proud of the result achieved by this untutored seaman on a mutinous whaling ship in the Pacific.

AN EXTRAORDINARY SURGICAL OPERATION

The San Francisco surgeon Elias Samuel Cooper had a Latin motto written over his bed: *Nulla dies sine linea*—"No day without a line," a phrase used by the ancient Greek painter Apelles to describe his utter dedication to his art. Cooper, too, believed in letting no day go to waste. An insatiable autodidact, he slept for only four hours a night and packed more into his forty years than many who live for twice as long. Not all of it was good: He was regularly embroiled in court cases, alienated many of his colleagues and was widely suspected of grave robbing in order to obtain cadavers for his anatomy classes. But he also founded the first medical school on the west coast of America, pioneered the use of chloroform and the caesarean section, and performed numerous operations of breathtaking audacity.

Of all his achievements, however, there was one that Cooper regarded with particular satisfaction, an operation so fraught that he described it unhesitatingly as the most difficult he ever performed. It was reported in an 1858 edition of *The Medical and Surgical Reporter* under a headline that was, if anything, an understatement:

1. *Extraordinary Surgical Operation.*

At the request of a committee of the San Francisco County Medico-Chirurgical Association, Dr. E. S. Cooper of that city has furnished them with a detailed account of an operation performed by him for the removal of a foreign body from beneath the heart!

In 1857, the idea of operating inside the chest was so terrifying as to be almost unthinkable. It was occasionally necessary when projectiles such as musket balls had penetrated the lungs, but only as a measure of last resort. It was inherently risky, since opening the chest would let air into the thoracic cavity, causing the lungs to collapse. This could quickly bring about respiratory failure, killing the patient by suffocation. And the location of this foreign object—underneath the heart—added another layer of difficulty to the operation. Many surgeons believed that even touching the heart could cause it to stop beating. The first procedure to treat a cardiac wound did not take place until 1896, partly because so many experts thought that manipulating the organ was virtually impossible.

> *Dr. Cooper does not tell us what length of time was consumed in performing his extraordinary operation, though he mentions that "at least three-quarters of an hour" were consumed in an exploration of the thoracic cavity by means of a sound* for the purpose of discovering the location of the foreign body. This may give the reader some idea of the entire length of time occupied in the operation.*

At a conservative estimate, it must have taken more than two hours. This is not exceptional by modern standards, but you haven't heard the half of it yet . . .

> *Mr. B. T. Beal, aged twenty-five, of Springfield, Tuolumne County, California, with some other young men, in a frolicsome mood, resolved to burst an old gun, and accordingly loaded it with about eighteen inches of powder, to which they connected a slow match and then endeavored to seek security by flight.*

"Guys, I'm in a frolicsome mood. Shall we blow up an old cannon?"

> *Unfortunately, a brisk wind blew up the powder with great rapidity, and the gun exploded before they had retreated far. A slug of iron had been driven into the gun as a temporary breech-pin, which, bursting out in the explosion, struck Mr. Beal in the left side below the armpit, fracturing the sixth rib,*

---

* Probe

entering the chest and lodging, as was afterwards found, be-
neath the heart upon the vertebral column, just to the right of
the descending aorta, where it had evidently remained from
the period of the injury, January 25, 1857, until it was re-
moved April 9, seventy-four days after.

This is a pretty extraordinary set of circumstances. The fact that the "slug of iron" had entered the man's chest without killing him outright is surprising—it might easily have destroyed any number of important structures, including major blood vessels or the heart itself. And goodness only knows how he managed to survive for two months afterward.

In a state of extreme prostration he was brought to the city,
having had frequent discharges of several ounces of purulent
matter at a time from the chest through the original wound.
The left lung had lost its function, probably less on account of
the violence done the lung at the time than from the subsequent
accumulation of pus in the chest, though he had bloody expecto-
ration for a few days. He came to my Infirmary on Mission
Street 8th of April, and during the night following had alarm-
ing symptoms of suffocation, so much so that I entertained most
serious apprehensions that he would not live till morning.

The surgeon would have preferred to let his patient "obtain rest from the fatigues of his journey" but became so alarmed by his condition that he decided to operate first thing the following day. Dr. Cooper was not a superstitious man, but as he prepared for surgery, he had a strange experience that he would later liken to a premonition. While selecting and laying out his instruments, he found himself drawn to an "awkward and ungainly" pair of forceps, an item designed for removing bladder stones and ill suited to the procedure he was about to perform. Without much thought, he slipped them into his pocket and went to the operating room to get on with the job.

Operation.—The patient being placed on the right side, an incision through the soft parts three inches long was made.

When the surgeon cut through the patient's muscles, he found that one rib was broken and already in a state of decay—no doubt caused by infection. He enlarged the incision so that it encompassed the original wound, and then had to pause to tie shut two or three arteries that had started to bleed.

The wound was now fully absterged,* after which an effort was made to find the breech-pin by using the probe. This failing, the incisions were lengthened and the ribs further exposed.

What has been described so far would not necessarily be out of place in a modern surgical case report. But here's the thing: This patient *was fully conscious.* Anesthesia was widely available by 1857, but the surgeon decided to do without. This may have been because of the danger of asphyxiation: Both chloroform and ether depress respiratory function, increasing the risk of sudden death.

A portion of the sixth rib, which was carious,† was now removed, and was followed by the discharge of about ten ounces of fluid resembling venous blood, contained in a cyst which was broken by the removal of the portion of the rib. A most extensive

---

* Wiped clean
† Decayed

but careful examination with the probe was now made in order to detect, if possible, the foreign body, yet to no purpose; but air having already been admitted into the chest I unhesitatingly removed portions of the fifth and seventh ribs, together with such an additional piece of the sixth as was necessary to make ample room to afford every facility for the further prosecution of the search.

Just put yourself in the patient's place for a moment. Wide awake, with a surgeon carving large chunks out of your ribs and having a good rummage inside your thorax.

Some very firm adventitious attachments were now broken up with the fingers, which gave exit to an immense amount of purulent matter—two quarts at least—which had been entirely disconnected with the fluid first discharged from the chest.*

A quite horrifying amount of pus: well over two liters.

The pleura had several large holes through it and was thickened to four or six times its natural state in some parts. The pulsations of the heart in the pericardium could be distinctly seen through these holes. Brandy was now administered freely to the patient who appeared to be rapidly sinking.

Given the experience the poor man was going through, this is hardly surprising. Brandy was here being administered as a

---

* Adhesions between adjacent structures, caused by scar tissue

stimulant, though in his situation, I suspect I'd be asking for something even stronger.

The left lung was found completely collapsed after the discharge of purulent matter. By giving brandy freely the patient soon began to revive, when the search for the foreign body was resumed. At this time the fingers could be placed upon different portions of the heart and feel its pulsations distinctly, but could obtain no clue to the location of the foreign body.

While not actually painful, the sensation of having your heart touched by a surgeon's fingers cannot be a pleasant one.

The patient now appeared almost completely exhausted. Brandy was given freely.

Only now (!) was anesthesia contemplated.

Chloroform was not administered at first, owing to the expected collapse of the left lung on the admission of air into the chest, but a considerable reaction taking place a limited quantity was now used, and the manipulations continued. A sound was introduced and the thoracic cavity explored for at least three-quarters of an hour before anything like a metallic touch could be recognized, and then it was so indistinct as to leave the matter doubtful.

From the description, it sounds as if the dose of chloroform was only enough to produce light sedation rather than full anesthesia. The surgeon now continued his epic search for the rogue piece of metal.

The space immediately above the diaphragm was considered the region in which the metal was most likely to be found; since the immense amount of suppuration which had taken place, it was thought might have dislodged, and gravitation carried it down to the bottom of the chest. The metal not being found here there was no longer any probable opinion to be formed as to its whereabouts, and to describe the difficulties of the search that followed would be difficult if not impossible.

In the annals of early surgery, there is virtually nothing to match this operation for complexity and sheer jeopardy. In an age before X-rays, finding a small foreign body that might be virtually anywhere in the chest cavity, without killing the patient, was a truly herculean task.

No one can have any just conception of the degree of patience required to do what was done, save the one who did it. This is not spoken boastingly, but it is simply the truth. It is sufficient to say that a general exploration of that side of the chest was made, and then it was taken by sections, occasionally passing through holes in the pleura, which latter appeared to have scarcely no normal relations to the surrounding structures, touching by lines the entire surface of the parts, and at last the sound appeared to encounter something of a metallic nature beneath the heart, but the pulsations of that organ were so strong against the instrument as to render it difficult to settle the matter definitely.

This is phenomenal stuff. Dr. Cooper was performing delicate manipulations, around a beating heart, that would not become a normal part of surgical practice for many decades.

At last, however, it became evident that the location of the iron was found, and I endeavored to move it out of its position with the point of the sound, in order to get it into a place more eligible for extraction by the forceps. I failed in this, and in manoeuvring the instrument finally lost the track by which the sound had first passed back of the heart to the metal, and it was during my efforts to recover this, and which was accomplished with the more difficulty owing to some membranes falling in the way, that I discovered the sound had in the first instance reached the metal by passing between the descending aorta and the apex of the heart.

Terrifying! Unknown to the surgeon, he had stuck his probe through the minute aperture between the largest blood vessel in the body and the heart itself. One slip and it was curtains for the patient. Dr. Cooper now tried to extract the metal object, but repeatedly failed to grab hold of it. Every instrument his assistant handed him was as ineffective as the last, until with a flash of inspiration he remembered the forceps in his pocket. They were precisely what he needed.

The metal being again found, the sound was steadily and strongly held in contact with it until a pair of long lithotomy forceps was thereby conducted to the spot and the breech-pin seized and extracted, which, however, was the work of several minutes, owing to the great difficulty in grasping it even after the forceps was made to touch it.

At last! It's exhausting just reading this; imagine how the patient felt. His protracted ordeal at an end, the wound was now dressed and he was taken back to a ward to rest. His recovery was long and arduous, but in early August, his condition was reported as follows:

The external wound has entirely cicatrized.* No cough nor pain in the left side—good appetite and all the functions of the system well performed. The left breast is somewhat sunken, but the upper lobe of that lung has recovered in a great degree its former action.

The left lung was almost destroyed by the injury and subsequent infection, so this represents an impressive recovery. Dr. Cooper ends his report with an endorsement of the California lifestyle so enthusiastic that the San Francisco tourist board might have used it on their advertisements:

His subsequent astonishing recovery is attributed to his great cheerfulness, good constitution, and to the effects of our unparalleled climate, in which it appears nearly impossible for a patient to die with almost any ordinary degree of injury, provided a reasonable share of attention is afterwards given him.

His recovery was indeed nothing short of astounding. Five years later it was reported that

He has since walked across the plains with a drove of cattle;—got married, and has a family.

Somehow, I doubt he dared hope for such a thing as he lay there awake on the operating table, with a surgeon holding his beating heart.

----

* Healed

5

REMARKABLE
RECOVERIES

THE HUNTERIAN MUSEUM of the Royal College of Surgeons in London is one of the world's great medical collections, a cathedral of glass jars containing organs and exotic species preserved in formaldehyde. It was founded in 1799 when the British government bought more than fifteen thousand anatomical specimens amassed by the celebrated surgeon John Hunter, who had died six years earlier, and has since been augmented by numerous curiosities, paintings and surgical instruments. In May 1941, a German incendiary bomb fell on the building, destroying the bulk of Hunter's original collection and some of the museum's most prized specimens. One of the artifacts lost forever that night was a partial human skeleton that in the nineteenth century had shared a pedestal with an ex-elephant. The bones were those of the late Thomas Tipple, who in his day had been something of a medical celebrity.

On the evening of June 13, 1812, Tipple went to see a friend in Stratford, a short distance east of London. He traveled in a gig, a light two-wheeled carriage pulled by a single horse. When he arrived, no groom was available to help him, so Tipple decided to unharness the animal himself. He had got no further than taking off the bridle before the horse started forward unexpectedly, driving one of the shafts of the vehicle straight through the left side of Tipple's chest. Such was the force involved that it emerged underneath his right armpit, pinning the unfortunate Tipple to the stable wall like an insect in a Victorian entomologist's collection. The first people on the scene found him still conscious, and he was able to help them remove the large wooden shaft that had completely impaled him.

To general amazement, Tipple walked up two flights of stairs unaided, and took off his own vest before going to bed. He survived for another eleven years, despite receiving the minimum of medical attention, which consisted mainly of having three pints of blood evacuated from an arm.* When he died in 1823, a postmortem established that the iron-tipped shaft had broken several of his ribs, almost certainly puncturing a lung in the process.

For much of the nineteenth century, the miraculous survival of Thomas Tipple was cited as an example of the astonishing resilience of the human frame. Life may be fragile, but there are plenty of tales from medical history that demonstrate that we can sometimes overcome even the most formidable injury. Many of these recoveries were attributable to the devotion or ingenuity of a conscientious doctor; some patients, however, may have got better despite, rather than thanks to, any treatment they received. Medicine is a field in which it is notoriously difficult to make a meaningful connection between cause and effect—a fact that has emboldened countless charlatans to make outrageous claims about the supposed efficacy of their particular brand of snake oil. One nineteenth-century

---

* Given that he was bleeding internally, this was the exact opposite of what should have happened.

doctor claimed that his patient's paralysis had disappeared when the ship he was traveling on was struck by lightning, while another reported that a train crash had cured one passenger of rheumatic fever. While such case reports may not be quite as compelling an advertisement for the wonders of medicine as their authors assumed, they are often a powerful affirmation of the human spirit.

THE WANDERING MUSKET BALL

Robert Fielding, the son of a Gloucestershire clergyman, was twenty-two and had just graduated from Oxford when the English Civil War began in 1642. A passionate Royalist, he joined the king's army and on September 20, 1643, took part in the First Battle of Newbury, at which Charles was defeated by the Parliamentarians. As well as being on the losing side, Fielding was seriously wounded, and for a time his survival seemed unlikely. Against the odds, he was able to resume his academic career at Oxford, at least until the victorious Roundheads ejected him from his college fellowship three years later. He was, however, readmitted as a student to study medicine, and in middle age became a prominent and much-loved physician in Gloucester, even being elected the city's mayor in 1670.

That he achieved any of this is pretty impressive, because he did so with a large slug of metal inside his head. In 1708, the *Philosophical Transactions* printed Dr. Fielding's own account of the battle-field injury that put it there.

VIII. *A Brief Narrative of the Shot of Dr.* Robert Fielding *with a Musket-Bullet, and its ſtrange manner of coming out of his Head, where it had lain near Thirty Years. Written by Himſelf.*

At the first Newberry fight, in the time of the late Civil Wars,
the doctor was shot by the right eye on the os petrosum* by the
orbit of the eye to the skull, which was likewise broke, with great
effusion of blood from the wound, mouth and nostrils. The sur-
geon carefully probing the wound for the discovery of the bullet,
but failing of his intention, on the third day after the shot
placed him horizontal to the sun; by which means depressing
the broken skull with the probe, he could feel the palpitation of
the brain, but could not discover the bullet.

It's no exaggeration to describe this procedure as brain surgery—
not much fun under battlefield conditions. For some time afterward, fragments of bone continued to emerge from various orifices,
an event always preceded by an odd symptom: His jaw became
locked shut.

When the doctor began to grow cold, his mouth closed up, and
so continued for the space of half a year till many fractures of
bones were come out of the wound, mouth and nostrils.

Bone fragments started to appear with horrific regularity. On the
plus side, he now had a startling new party trick:

Afterwards, whensoever a scale of bone was to come out his
mouth would close, insomuch that several years afterwards he
prognosticated to some friends that a bone was then coming out,
which continued so for six or seven weeks, at which time finding
an itching in the orifice of the wound, with his finger he felt a

---

* One of the bones of the skull

bone, upon which he made known to some friends then present, that they should see him open his mouth, and taking out a bone no bigger than a pin's head, he immediately opened his mouth.

Why was the doctor unable to open his mouth, and why did removing a bone fragment relieve the condition? It seems likely that the wound was near the mandibular nerve, which controls the four muscles responsible for biting and chewing. If a splinter of bone was pressing on this nerve, it could cause temporary paralysis, relieved only once the pressure had been removed. A year after the original injury, the wound finally healed. But there was still no sign of the musket ball—much to Dr. Fielding's chagrin.

After this, for the space of ten years, or more, a flux of sanious matter issued out of the right nostril, and then ceasing there, it flowed from the left nostril for some years.

Sanious describes a thin watery liquid. This seems likely to have been cerebrospinal fluid (CSF)—the liquid that cushions the brain against injury. CSF leaks are often the consequence of an injury to the dura, the membrane surrounding the brain.

At length, for the space of two years, or thereabouts, upon riding, the doctor would sometimes find a pain on the left side about the almonds of the ear, which he attributed to cold, but more especially after riding in a cold dark night, which occasioned a kind of deafness too.

The "almonds of the ear" are the tonsils—the name by which they were known to non-medics in the seventeenth century.

*And having stopped his ear with wool to recover his hearing,
one day, either writing or reading, suddenly an huff* came in
the ear, which made him start, and in the manner not to be
expressed, unless you can imagine a vacuum; this happened
about March or April 1670. Upon this all that side of the cheek
hung loose as though paralytic, and under the ear might be felt
a hard knob.*

Though the facial paralysis sounds a bit like a stroke, it was probably something more benign. The compression of another nerve[†] by
a bone fragment (or by the elusive musket ball) would cause similar
symptoms.

*After this, tumour upon tumour appeared on that side under
the jawbone, which occasioned his consulting some physicians,
two at one time, one of which suspected the bullet, which, considering the shot, they thought not credible. At length the tumours coming to the throat, if he held up his head a little, it
seemed as if one with a hook did pull down the jawbone; and if
anything touched the throat, it was as painful as if pricked
with a handful of needles; being at last persuaded to make some
applications, a small hole appeared, after that another, and a
third part near the pomum adami;[‡] by these the bullet was discovered, and cut out in August 1672.*

Amazing. Dr. Fielding had been shot almost thirty years earlier,
and it took all this time for the musket ball to migrate—somehow—
from the upper part of his skull to his throat, where it was finally

---

* A gust or puff of wind
† Most likely cranial nerve VII, also known as the facial nerve
‡ Adam's apple

extracted. Miraculously, he seems not to have been even slightly impaired by the presence of this piece of lead in his skull, and was still well enough to write about it more than six decades after the original injury.

THE MILLER'S TALE

The Isle of Dogs, a large peninsula on the north bank of the Thames, is an area of London not generally known for its bucolic charm. The skyscrapers of Canary Wharf house one of Europe's largest financial centers, while remnants of the heavy industry that once supported the local economy still peek out from between expensive apartment blocks. But until the late eighteenth century, the area was sparsely populated farmland, the only significant buildings a line of windmills built on the western flood defenses* to take advantage of the stiff breezes coming off the river.

In 1737, a worker at one of these mills had an accident so astounding that he became a local celebrity. Prints of Samuel Wood's likeness were sold in taverns and bookshops, and his case was still being quoted in scientific journals well over a century later. The surgeon who treated him, John Belchier, described what had happened to his famous patient at a meeting of the Royal Society a few months later:

> V. *An Account of the* Man *whofe* Arm *with the* Shoulder-blade *was torn off by a* Mill, *the* 15th *of* Auguft 1737. *by* Mr. John Belchier, *F. R. S. Surgeon to* Guy's *Hofpital.*

---

* An area known ever since as Millwall

Samuel Wood, about 26 years of age, being at work in one of the
mills near the Isle of Dogs, over-against* Deptford, and going
to fetch a sack of corn from the farther part of the mill in order
to convey it up into the hopper, carelessly took with him a rope,
at the end of which was a slipknot which he had put round his
wrist; and passing by one of the large wheels, the cogs of it
caught hold of the rope, and he not being able to disengage his
hand instantly, was drawn towards the wheel and raised off
the ground, till his body being checked by the beam which sup-
ports the axis of the wheel, his arm with the shoulder-blade
was separated from it.

Sounds excruciating. At least, that's what you'd think.

At the time the accident happened, he says he was not sensible
of any pain, but only felt a tingling about the wound, and be-
ing a good deal surprised, did not know that his arm was torn
off till he saw it in the wheel.

Put yourself in Samuel Wood's shoes for a minute: Imagine spying
an arm stuck in a piece of machinery and only then realizing that it
is yours.

When he was a little recovered, he came down a narrow ladder
to the first floor of the mill, where his brother was, who seeing
his condition, ran downstairs immediately out of the mill to a
house adjacent to the next mill, which is about a hundred yards
distant from the place where the accident happened, and
alarmed the inhabitants with what had happened to his

---

* Opposite

brother; but before they could get out of the house to his assistance, the poor man had walked by himself to within about ten yards of the house, where, being quite spent by the great effusion of blood, he fainted away and lay on the ground; they immediately took him up, and carried him into the house, and strewed a large quantity of loaf-sugar powdered into the wound in order to stop the blood till they could have the assistance of a surgeon, whom they sent instantly for to Limehouse.

Sugar was generally sold in conical loaves in the eighteenth century and would have to be broken down and powdered by hand before use. It may seem strange to put it on a wound, but it was often used in such scenarios, and is still a common remedy in many developing countries. There has even been some recent interest in the use of sugar as a possible antimicrobial agent in the management of wounds.

But the messenger being very much frighted, could not give the surgeon a clear idea of the accident, so that when he came to see the condition the man was in, he had no dressings with him for an accident of that kind; but had brought with him an apparatus for a broken arm, which he understood by what he could learn from the messenger to be the case.

Equipment that was certainly inadequate for the task in hand.

However, he sent home for proper dressings, and when he came to examine particularly into the wound, in order to secure the large blood vessels, there was not the least appearance of any, nor any effusion of blood; so having first brought the fleshy parts of the wound as near together as he could by means of a

needle and ligature, he dressed him up with a warm digestive,*
and applied a proper bandage.

The next morning, the surgeon checked the wound for bleeding,
and was surprised to find none. After changing the dressing, he
sent Samuel Wood to St. Thomas's Hospital so that he could be
kept under close observation, in the care of a surgeon called James
Ferne.

He was constantly attended, in expectation of a haemorrhage
of blood from the subclavian artery; but there being no appear-
ance of fresh bleeding, it was not thought proper to remove the
dressings during the space of four days, when Mr Ferne opened
the wound, at which time likewise there was not the least ap-
pearance of any blood vessels; so he dressed him up again, and
in about two months' time the cure was entirely completed.

The accidental amputation was evidently a neat job, leaving plenty
of skin and muscle to heal over the wound. When they examined
the severed limb, the doctors found the shoulder blade and both
bones of the forearm had been broken . . .

. . . but whether these bones were fractured before the arm was
torn off, the man cannot possibly judge.

The poor man had had his arm and shoulder blade ripped off by
industrial machinery. It seems fairly safe to assume that the triple
fracture in that arm was caused by the accident rather than being a
freak coincidence.

-----

* An ointment intended to promote wound healing

But why hadn't he bled to death? A major blood vessel, the sub-clavian artery, had been severed as a result of the injury. In normal circumstances, this would have produced copious bleeding, per-haps enough to kill him in under an hour. But somehow this had not happened. The surgeon concluded that the tissues around the artery had compressed it, acting as a tourniquet and preventing any loss of blood.

Mr. Belchier was well aware that his story might not be believed: Medical tall tales of dubious provenance were often reported with-out a shred of supporting evidence. So he went to some trouble to ensure that there was no doubt about this one.

As this case is so very singular and so remarkable that no history can furnish us with any instance similar to it, in order to give a particular account of it, besides visiting the man frequently, from his first admittance into the hospital, and getting from him what information he was capable of giving me, I went myself two days ago to the mill where the accident happened, and en-quired into every particular circumstance relating to the fact.

But that wasn't all. With a theatrical flourish, Mr. Belchier revealed to the assembled dignitaries that he had brought a special guest and an unusual prop with him:

And for the further satisfaction of the Society, I have brought the man himself, and likewise the arm, just as 'twas torn from his body, which has been kept in spirits ever since the accident happened.

Talk about a showstopper! In the later editions of his *Anatomy of the Human Body*, the eighteenth-century surgeon William

Cheselden included a handsome engraving of Samuel Wood, the miller gazing wistfully toward a bucolic landscape in which a windmill can be glimpsed just above the tree line. It's a romantic vision, if one ignores the object dominating the foreground: his severed arm, its nerves and tendons laid bare by the brutal accident that he was so lucky to survive.

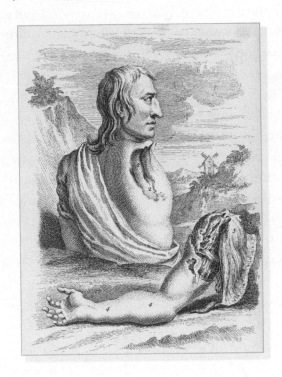

IN ONE SIDE AND OUT THE OTHER

When Dr. Henry Yates Carter submitted three articles to the *Medical Facts and Observations* in 1795, he described himself as a "surgeon at Kettley, near Wellington, in Shropshire." This makes him sound like a humble country doctor, but it would be more accurate to describe him as a globe-trotting adventurer. Born in London, he crossed the Atlantic after the death of his parents to take up an apprenticeship with an uncle in Philadelphia. He served as a battlefield surgeon during the War of Independence, then joined the Royal Navy and saw action on both sides of the Atlantic. In 1782, he was the ship's surgeon of HMS *Formidable*, Admiral Rodney's flagship, at the Battle of the Saintes—a famous engagement during which the British beat off a planned invasion of the Caribbean by French and Spanish forces. He retired to practice medicine in England for a few years, finally emigrating to Pennsylvania, where he died in 1849, a few months short of his hundredth birthday.

The cases he sent to the London journal were an unusual mixture of the rustic and the revolutionary. One involved an accident with a waterwheel, another a man whose foot had been run over by a horse and cart. But perhaps the pick of the bunch is this story from his days on the battlefields of America, almost twenty years earlier:

IV. *Cafe of a Gun-Shot Wound of the Head. By the fame.*

A Hessian grenadier, aged between thirty and forty years, being one of a detachment sent to reduce a fort on the banks of the Delaware, in the act of levelling his piece,* received a ball (grape shot) on that part of the os frontis† which forms the external canthus‡ of the eye. The ball making its passage through the head, came out under and rather behind the opposite ear, as in the annexed plate.

---

* i.e., raising his musket to fire it
† The frontal bone, which makes up the forehead and the upper part of the eye sockets
‡ The corner of the eye nearest the temple

Hessians were German soldiers who were engaged to fight for the British in the War of Independence, to the fury of many American patriots. Dr. Yates's mention of the Delaware gives good grounds for thinking that this soldier was injured in December 1776 at the Battle of Trenton, in which the Hessians played a major role. The path taken by the shot (from "a" to "b") is quite clear in the accompanying illustration:

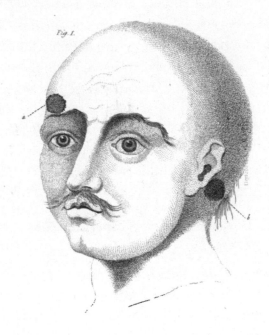

What were the immediate effects upon the receipt of the injury I am not able to say, not being immediately upon the spot; but he appeared, when brought to the regimental hospital, to have a perfect recollection of every circumstance that had occurred to him, except only for a short time after he fell. He complained of little pain, and did not appear to have lost so much blood as

might have been expected. The ball being a spent one, had much splintered the cranium, both at its entrance and exit; and was found in the folds of his coat collar.

Much better to find it there than know it is still inside your brain, I suppose.

The wounds being cleansed, and the splinters of bone removed as far as was practicable from about the external parts, suitable dressings were applied; and his pulse being full, he was let blood; after which he took twenty-five drops of tincture of opium. The next day he had a sense of heaviness over his eyes, and observed that objects did not appear to him so brilliant as usual; towards the evening he complained of nausea and thirst.

Given what had just happened to him, observing that objects "do not appear so brilliant as usual" seems a mild symptom to have to put up with. Over the next few days, the treatment prescribed for the patient—bizarrely, you might think, but quite routinely for the time—concentrated on his bowels: He was given regular clysters, or enemas.

On the third day he complained of pain of his head, accompanied with drowsiness; and, at intervals, of a weakness of his extremities. As the clysters had failed to procure a sufficient discharge of faeces, he was directed to take three grains of calomel and fifteen grains of powder of jalap, which operated well, and procured an alleviation of the symptoms just now mentioned. His eyes were but slightly inflamed, and he complained of but little pain in that on the affected side.

On the sixth day, there was "a pretty good discharge of matter from the wound"—and no doubt from his bowels as well—and his condition began to improve.

> *Splinters of bone that had been driven in at the superior wound by the ball came away from the dependent orifice at almost every dressing (which was twice a day) for several days.*

These bone fragments were pieces of his forehead and eye socket, but they were emerging from a wound behind his ear! Curiouser and curiouser.

> *The nausea, headache, weakness of his limbs, thirst, and every symptom of fever, gradually vanished; the superior orifice filled up with new granulations, and cicatrized firmly; and in about ten weeks there remained nothing more necessary than a superficial dressing to the inferior opening near the ear.*

In little more than two months, the wound had healed. And here's the amazing thing: The man made a full recovery.

> *I did not see this man after he had actually left off every application to the affected part; but from the condition of the wound, and the patient's health and vigour, I have not any room to doubt, that in a few days after I last saw him he was capable of returning to his duty.*

When you consider the mess that piece of grapeshot must have made in its progress from one side of his head to the other, it's a marvel that he made it out of his sickbed, let alone back to the front line.

A BAYONET THROUGH THE HEAD

Not even Alexandre Dumas could have invented a hero as improbably courageous, gallant and talented as Urbain-Jean Fardeau. By turns a teacher, priest, soldier and surgeon, he excelled in every occupation he tried. Combining his medical studies with a swashbuckling career in the French Revolutionary Army, he so distinguished himself with the sword that he was one of the first recipients of the Légion d'honneur in 1802. An hour after it was presented to him by Napoleon Bonaparte in a splendid ceremony near Boulogne, Fardeau dived into a churning sea (pausing only to kiss the insignia freshly pinned on his tunic by the emperor) and swam out to a boat that had got into difficulties, saving more than 150 lives.

During the War of the Fourth Coalition, Fardeau accompanied Napoleon's armies in their campaign in Eastern Europe, and was present at the Battle of Pułtusk on December 26, 1806, an encounter that took place in the bitter cold of the Polish winter. While there, he witnessed an unusual incident, which he later narrated to a meeting of the Medical Society of Paris:

> *Observation sur une plaie de tête faite par une bayonnette lancée par un boulet, par M. FARDEAU, ex-chirurgien d'armée, membre de la Légion d'honneur, etc.*
> Lue à la Société le 20 juin 1809.

A soldier named Malva, a voltigeur from my regiment, was wounded in the head by a bayonet which had been unmounted and propelled by a cannonball.

The *voltigeurs* were specialist light infantry soldiers. Their name means literally "vaulters": It was originally intended that they should travel into battle by leaping onto the rump of a passing cavalry horse, before sliding lightly to the ground to fight on foot.* The soldier named Malva had discovered a notably unlucky way to get injured. It seems that the bayonet, while still mounted to a rifle, had been struck by a cannonball and dislodged, turning it into a lethal missile. Its velocity must have been tremendous, so one would expect it to do a huge amount of damage.

> *The* voltigeur *was struck on the right temple, two fingers' breadth beyond the angle of the orbit and a little above it. The bayonet (which was between 12 and 14 inches long) passed up to the hilt, from the front towards the back, and from above downwards, so as to traverse the maxillary sinus on the opposite side, and projected five inches.*

The maxillary sinus is one of the cavities of the skull, beneath the cheekbone. It is also known by the rather more poetic name "antrum of Highmore," which sounds more like a Scottish aristocrat than an anatomical feature. The bayonet had therefore passed right through the skull, entering the right temple and exiting the left cheek, with no less than five inches of blade visible beyond the exit wound. This situation might be described as less than ideal.

> *The man was knocked down, but did not lose consciousness. He made several ineffectual efforts to pull the bayonet out, and two*

---

* This scheme didn't last long, as everybody involved soon realized it was a deeply silly idea.

comrades, one holding the head, while the other tugged at the weapon, also failed.

After this touching scene, which rather puts me in mind of two hungry birds tugging at the same worm, the soldiers admitted defeat and took their comrade to see the regimental surgeon.

The poor wounded man came to me leaning on the arms of two fellow-soldiers. I endeavoured with the assistance of a soldier to pull out the bayonet, but it seemed to me as if fixed in a wall. The soldier who helped me told the patient to lie down on his side, put his foot on the man's head, and with both hands heaved out the bayonet; a considerable haemorrhage immediately followed, the blood pouring out violently and abundantly.

A surgical procedure that entails putting your foot on the patient's head is rarely a subtle one. Nor indeed sensible, in this case: Today a doctor would want to be pretty sure what structures the bayonet had damaged, and where it lay in relation to the blood vessels, before attempting to remove it. But we must make allowances for the exigencies of battlefield medicine.

For the first time Malva felt unwell; I thought he would die, so left him to bandage other casualties. After twenty minutes he revived, saying that he was much better, and I then dressed his wound. We were in the snow, and it was bitterly cold; I wrapped the whole of his head well in charpie and bandages.

Charpie was a material used for surgical dressings, consisting of thin strips of linen unraveled into threads.

> *He set off for Warsaw with another wounded soldier; he trav-*
> *elled on foot, on horseback, in a cart from barn to barn, and*
> *often from wood to wood, and reached Warsaw in six days,*
> *having travelled 20 leagues.* I met him again three months*
> *later in hospital, perfectly recovered. He had lost his sight on*
> *the right side: the eye and lid had retained their form and mo-*
> *bility, but the iris remained much dilated and immovable.*

Which is not a bad outcome, if you've recently had a bayonet through your head. At this point the soldier Malva drops out of the historical record, although we know plenty more about M. Fardeau. After leaving the army, he returned to his hometown of Saumur and became a celebrated ophthalmic surgeon, tending to the poor and generally living a blameless and philanthropic life. Nobody seems to have had a bad word to say about him; in fact, the only reason Dumas never wrote a book about Urbain-Jean Fardeau may be that he was just too damn nice.

AN INTERESTING AND REMARKABLE ACCIDENT

This is one of those cases that at first reading seems inherently unlikely—but, bizarre as it sounds, has a perfectly rational medical explanation. It took place in the 1830s but was only reported in any detail three-quarters of a century later. This account was written by Dr. Roswell Park, an American pioneer of neurosurgery who also founded the first institution in the world to be dedicated solely to cancer research.† Dr. Park had stumbled across the story a long

---

* About seventy miles
† Created in 1898 as the Pathological Laboratory of the University of Buffalo, it is now known as Roswell Park Comprehensive Cancer Center.

time earlier, and was so astonished by what he read that he decided
to investigate further.

**Fracture of the Atlas : Separation of a Fragment, and Its
Subsequent Extrusion Through the Mouth**

The Unique Case of Dr. James P. White

Reported by ROSWELL PARK

---

*There came into my possession some twenty years ago, perhaps
longer, the subjoined statements regarding the nature of a very
unusual accident, with still rarer sequels, which befell Dr.
James P. White, one of the founders of the Buffalo General
Hospital, during the year 1837.*

James Platt White was an influential gynecologist, a founding professor of the University of Buffalo and a prominent member of Buffalo
society in the mid-nineteenth century. He was the first American
medic to conduct obstetric demonstrations with real patients, allowing his students to listen to the fetal heart and examine the birth canal
as labor advanced. This practice was already widespread in Europe,
but American students were still expected to learn their midwifery
from textbooks and mannequins, and his innovation caused great
controversy among those who believed such practices indecent.

*In December of that year something happened to the stagecoach
in which he was riding, near Batavia, and he was violently
thrown, and in such a way as to seriously injure his head and
neck. I have not been able to learn any of the details either of
the event or of his subsequent symptoms.*

All we know thus far is that Dr. White injured his head and neck in
a stagecoach accident. So far, so unremarkable; and of the next six

weeks of his life nothing is known. But after that, something truly extraordinary happened to him: He coughed up part of his own spine.

Well, it's better than coughing up somebody else's.

This surprising occurrence was reported in a short statement that appeared in *The Medical News* in 1886. It was written by Joseph Pancoast, a leading surgeon of the day and therefore (one would hope) a trustworthy source. Dr. Pancoast was happy to confirm that this unlikely incident had taken place, and had even seen the portion of Dr. White's spine, which he described as

> *A front segment of the atlas vertebra, a little more than an inch on the superior margin, a little less below, with the facette which received the odontoid process.*

The atlas vertebra, also known as C1, is the topmost bone of the spine. It is named after Atlas, the Titan who in Greek mythology supported the sky on his shoulders. It's a feature of crucial importance since it protects part of the brainstem, which among other things regulates the heart rate and respiration. The mobility of the C1 vertebra also allows us to turn our heads and nod. The odontoid process or peg is a protuberance from C2, the second vertebra of the neck. The *facette* (now usually spelled *facet*) is the joint between the two vertebrae.

This chunk of bone was not the entire vertebra but a large portion of it. It seems that Dr. White had retained just enough of the bone to protect a critical part of his spinal cord from potentially fatal injury.

> *This bone, in possession of Professor Pattison, I repeatedly saw and carefully examined; he exhibited it to his class, and it was mislaid or lost.*

What a shame! It would have been quite an artifact.

> *The bone was in our possession in 1838-39-40, or thereabouts. I then understood and believed (since confirmed by conversation with Professor White) that it came from his throat, coming out through the mouth as a consequence of ulceration; the result of an accident while riding in a stagecoach on the morning of December 17th, 1837. The bone was discharged at the expiration of forty-five days after receipt of the injury.*

If there was ulceration at the back of the throat, it must have hurt like hell. There are very few comparable cases on record, but in all of them, the patient had great difficulty eating or drinking, was in severe pain and confined to bed. But who cares about mere agony? Can you imagine anything worse than suddenly "discharging" a large piece of your spine through your mouth? Writing seventy-five years after the nightmarish event, Roswell Park observes:

> *Of his condition during the forty five days previous to the extrusion of the fragment there is no account, neither is there of the time elapsing before his restoration to his usual activity; but inasmuch as he died in 1881, having passed the subsequent part of his life in a most active professional career, it is legitimate to conclude that he suffered little, if at all, from the consequences of his injury.*

He didn't escape its effects entirely: According to one obituary, the loss of his vertebra left him unable to turn his head.

In 2005, this case prompted an article by an eminent orthopedic surgeon working at White's old hospital in Buffalo, Eugene Mindell. After considering all the available evidence, Mindell concluded that White had suffered an injury known as a Jefferson fracture,* in which the atlas vertebra is shattered by a sharp impact. A few fragments of bone burst through the wall of the pharynx, causing an open wound that resulted in an infection of the exposed portion of vertebra. Eventually, the infection caused necrosis, when the dead portion of bone (known technically as a sequestrum) had come free and been coughed up (yuck). Finally, scar tissue had formed (or the two adjacent vertebrae C1 and C2 fused together) and the wound healed.

Dr. White was so little affected that he was able to return to work and live a normal life for more than thirty years afterward. In 1886, *The Medical News* described his injury as "an interesting and remarkable accident," a description that barely does it justice.

THE LUCKY PRUSSIAN

Maximilian Joseph von Chelius was a prominent nineteenth-century German surgeon who had a significant influence right across Europe. His lectures were frequently quoted in the London and Edinburgh journals, and his textbook *Handbuch der Chirurgie*, translated into English as *A System of Surgery*, was widely used.

In a chapter devoted to chest injuries, Chelius gives one particularly unusual case history, which had been sent to him by a friend

---

* Named after the British neurosurgeon Geoffrey Jefferson, who described the injury in an article published in 1919. The first case he encountered was that of an RAF pilot who had flown through a bank of telegraph wires at 120 miles per hour and somehow survived with little more than a sore neck.

in London, a Fellow of the Royal College of Surgeons called John
Goldwyer Andrews:*

IV.—OF WOUNDS OF THE CHEST.

*J.T., aged nineteen years, a Prussian sailor, whilst engaged in
lowering the trysail-mast, the rope supporting it gave way,
and he was transfixed by its bolt to the deck.*

On nineteenth-century ships, the trysail was a small sail that was
hoisted on a boom attached to the base of the mainmast. In a footnote,
Chelius explains that this "trysail-mast" was thirty-five feet long and
two feet in circumference, with a five-inch metal bolt at one end.

*At the time of the accident the mast had been lowered to within
about six feet of the deck; the man raised his arms to lay hold of
and guide the bolt into its proper place, when at the moment
the suspending rope slipped or broke, and the mast dropping
perpendicularly, fell on his chest.*

A thirty-five-foot mast of oak or pine would have been a fearsomely
heavy object. Oh, and did I mention that it had a five-inch metal
spike at the end?

*It knocked him down on his back, and the bolt passing through
his chest, pinned him to the deck, which it penetrated to the
depth of an inch, so that his chest must have been compressed,
from before backwards, to a space not exceeding four inches.*

---

* When he died in 1849, *The Lancet*'s obituary said of Mr. Andrews that he had "not
contributed anything to the advancement of medical or surgical knowledge, but was a
great patron of the fine arts." Which seems a bit harsh.

Four inches is about ten centimeters. Try to visualize that: The sailor's chest and its contents were crushed to a fraction of their usual depth.

Some time elapsed before the bolt could be drawn out, and he was then carried to the hospital.

There is no mention of how the bolt was removed—but it was preserved as a curiosity and later put on display in the Hunterian Museum, the anatomical collections of the Royal College of Surgeons.

Feb. 25, 1831: On his admission, 10 am, the countenance was livid, the breathing excessively distressed; small quantities of frothy blood were occasionally spat up, the pulse intermitting; and for some time after his admission, these symptoms increased, threatening almost immediate suffocation.

The "frothy blood" was an indication of bleeding within the lung, which had evidently been punctured by the iron bolt. It goes without saying that this was a life-threatening injury.

The bolt had entered the chest, between the fourth and fifth ribs of the left side, about an inch and a half from the middle of the breast-bone, passed obliquely downwards and outwards, and came out between the eleventh and twelfth ribs, four inches from the left side of the spine.

The chest was, the surgeon noted, "flattened" on one side, and damage to the rib cage had left the heart dangerously vulnerable. But this was not all:

In addition to this hurt, the scalp on the right side was consid-
erably lacerated, extending from the frontal to the lower part
of the occipital bone, and exposing a great part of the temporal
muscle. The lower jaw was also badly fractured.

The head wound, which was significant but not life-threatening, could be cleaned and bandaged, but in the 1830s, there was virtually nothing a surgeon could do for such a serious chest injury, except wait and hope that it was survivable.

A pledget* of lint was applied over the wound, and fastened
with adhesive straps, but nothing more was done, and two
hours after his admission the more urgent symptoms of suffoca-
tion had subsided, and he rallied a little.

The sailor passed a restless night, but to his doctors' relief, he was still alive the next morning. The therapeutic regime they adopted was orthodox for the time: It involved frequent applications of leeches, laxatives to purge the bowels and a bland diet of milk, arrowroot and powdered biscuits. Opium was frequently administered to ease his pain. His recovery was slow, but a month after the accident, he was reported to be doing well and living on blancmange and coffee. By the end of April, he was also "allowed table-beer and half a chicken daily," which sounds rather more appetizing. On May 25—some three months after the accident—he was finally convalescent, and well enough to leave the hospital.

This case also appears in a book by George Guthrie, a British surgeon who was one of Europe's leading experts on chest injuries. In his monograph *On Wounds and Injuries of the Chest* (1848),

---

* Wad

Guthrie records his amazement that the patient's symptoms had been so mild:

> *The quantity of blood spat up did not exceed that commonly coughed up in broken ribs. The discharge of pus from the wounds, till they had healed, was very trifling. The pulsation of the heart was very violent, distinctly raising the bedclothes. He lost about eighty ounces of blood from the arm, and had three hundred leeches applied at different times.*

The amount of blood (slightly more than four pints) taken directly from his veins is nothing too dramatic over the course of three months, but three hundred leeches must have added considerably to this total. The loss of so much of the red stuff cannot have done much for his complexion.

Ten years after the accident, Mr. Guthrie was invited to examine the patient for himself.

> *He was in good health; the breathing of the side injured good; the action of the heart violent, but not irregular. The depression made by the bolt and its cicatrix* was so directly over the great vessels, that it must have passed between them, pushing them aside, constituting altogether one of the most remarkable cases on record.*

Now, that really *is* extraordinary. The great vessels are the aorta and pulmonary artery, which are so closely entwined just above the heart that it's barely possible to get a cigarette paper between them, let alone a metal bolt.

---

* Scar

It was owing perhaps to the end of the bolt being blunt, and the great force, from the weight of the yard with which it was driven through, that the lung was but little injured.

Guthrie's suggestion seems quite sensible. His point is that when the human body is impaled, a blunt object sometimes does less damage than a sharp one, because rather than pierce the internal organs, it simply pushes them aside. Guthrie was speaking from experience—and he had made a careful study of similar injuries that seemed to bear out this theory.

But what of this patient's later career? After being pinned to the deck of a ship, you'd think he might have tried something less dangerous. But not a bit of it.

He recovered his health perfectly; first went into service as a footman, but returned to the sea, and was twice shipwrecked, and saved his life by swimming a considerable distance. In 1841 he was well, and went on a voyage to the West Indies.

At least nobody could accuse him of being risk-averse.

A CASE FOR DR. COFFIN

In 1837, a teenager from Gaspé in eastern Canada tripped in his parents' lawn and fell on a tool he was carrying. There was no great drama: The wound didn't bleed much, and after some basic first aid administered by his brother, he was able to walk back home for dinner.

It doesn't sound like much of a story—except that the tool was a scythe, and it went in one side of the boy's chest and out the other.

It caused a great sensation on both sides of the Atlantic when the details were first published some twelve years later, in a short-lived Canadian periodical, *The British American Journal of Medical and Physical Science.** The tale sounded so fantastic that the editor agreed to print it only after receiving evidence from three reliable witnesses, two of them doctors.

ART. LXXIII.—LATERAL TRANSFIXTURE OF THE CHEST BY A SCYTHE BLADE FOLLOWED BY COMPLETE RECOVERY, WITH REMARKS:
By E. Q. SEWELL, M. D., EDINBURGH,
Licentiate Royal College of Surgeons, Edinburgh, Member Royal Medical Society, &c.

The first on the scene, however, was not a medical man but a local justice of the peace, J. D. McConnell:

In the year 1837 Master James Boyle, a youth of about 18 years of age, had been mowing the lawn in the vicinity of his father's house, in company with his younger brother, and as is the custom, before going to dinner, he had taken the scythe off the snaith or handle, for the purpose of carrying it, in order to have it sharpened. As he walked homewards, a distance of about a few hundred yards, he happened to step on a log of wood, when his foot slipped and he fell upon the scythe blade, which entered his chest under the right armpit and the point appeared under the left. The hapless youth lay still with the deadly instrument in his breast until his brother, who displayed inimitable presence of mind, drew it slowly out, observing with much caution, as he did so, the curvature of the blade.

---

* Its founder, Archibald Hall, was terrible at coming up with snappy titles: In a later incarnation, the journal became known as *The British American Journal Devoted to the Advancement of Medical and Physical Sciences in the British-American Provinces.*

The effusion of blood which followed was not so great as might have been expected, and with his brother's aid he walked home.

The family would have preferred to summon a doctor, but in Gaspé, a tiny and remote coastal community at the easternmost tip of Quebec, that was not an option. A footnote explains:

> *There was no medical man resident in that vicinity when this occurrence took place. Frederick Coffin, a whaler, commonly called "Dr. Coffin"...*

A name that cannot have filled his patients with confidence.

> *... who generally lends a hand at bleeding, drawing teeth, and other similar services, has been very successful in his attempts at relieving the distressed. Under his care, the youth continued slowly to improve.*

A couple of days after the accident, a Royal Navy ship, HMS *Sappho*, happened to drop anchor in Gaspé Bay. A stroke of luck, for on board were no fewer than three medics.

> *I lost no time in making the case known to the surgeon of the ship, Mr. Thomson, who directed assistant surgeon Sproule to examine the patient, and to render any assistance that might be practicable, which that gentleman immediately did. I remember his remarking that the absence of bloody expectoration was a favourable symptom.*

Coughing up blood would have suggested an injury to the lung, an eventuality the boy seems to have escaped.

As the accident and its unexpected results appeared to me an inscrutable act of Providence, I deemed it desirable that Dr. Sproule should communicate to me by letter his opinion of the case.

The naval surgeon found that the point of the scythe had entered the boy's armpit, making a wound about 3 inches (7.5 cm) long between the third and fourth ribs on his right side. It had then passed horizontally through the chest before emerging at the same point on his left side. Dr. Sproule was mightily impressed:

Considering the situation of the wound, and the instrument by which it was made, I consider it a most miraculous escape, which I can only account for by saying that the back of the blade was directed towards the large blood vessels, and thereby protected them. Had the edge been otherwise directed, I have no doubt but that the consequences would have been immediately fatal.

Miraculous is not too strong a word. The symptoms were so mild that the scythe must somehow have avoided the major organs. Even so, it seems unlikely that a blade taking that course through the chest could have missed the pleura, the sac around the lungs. The author of the report, Dr. Sewell, suggests that the boy suffered a collapsed lung as air rushed into the thorax through the wound— but the puncture was so small that when the blade was removed, it sealed spontaneously, allowing the lung to reinflate. Whether or not this was precisely what happened, there's no doubt that he was very lucky.

It only remains to add, that Master James Boyle is, at present, a robust and vigorous man, and without any local complaint.

His pursuit is chiefly that of his father, a whaler, and his domicile is up the south-west branch of Gaspé Bay, in the district of Gaspé, Lower Canada.

A rare example of a Coffin saving a patient from an early grave.

THE HEALING POWER OF NATURE

At the annual meeting of the Provincial Medical and Surgical Association in August 1844, a doctor from Newport Pagnell in Buckinghamshire, Edward Daniell, presented this unusual case. He prefaced his account with the observation that it would "perhaps be interesting more from its novelty than for its value in a surgical point of view." He wasn't just being modest: As it turns out, his involvement in the proceedings was virtually nil.

EXTRAORDINARY CASE OF GUN-SHOT WOUND, WHERE THE CHARGE PASSED FROM THE NAVEL TO THE BACK, WITHOUT FATAL CONSEQUENCES.

By EDWARD DANIELL, ESQ., Newport Pagnel.

John Smith, a fisherman, aged about 25 years, went out on a Sunday morning in the winter of 1837 with two companions. One of these persons possessed a gun, which was so constructed that it could be taken to pieces and stowed in the pocket. I am not prepared to say whether these gentlemen designed a trespass on the game-laws, or whether their predatory excursions had only reference to those minor bipeds, which the legislature have considered too insignificant for their especial protection.

The "minor bipeds" alluded to by Mr. Daniell were any birds not covered by the Game Act of 1831, which made it illegal to shoot grouse, pheasant, partridge or wild chicken without a license. Theoretically, John Smith could have been shooting any other edible species such as pigeon, duck or even rooks quite legitimately—but even then, he would have needed the permission of the landowner.

> *I opine, however, that any wild animal capable of yielding a Sunday's dinner would have been in great jeopardy had it been luckless enough to cross their path at that time.*

Only professional etiquette prevents Mr. Daniell from calling his patient what he surely was: a poacher.

> *Certain it is they themselves felt that their pursuit was lawless, for they hastily took their weapon to pieces, on observing the owner of the fields approaching them. In re-adjusting it a second time the stock was not in perfect apposition, and the wiseacre* whose business it was to render the weapon fireworthy, observing this defect, sought to remedy it by striking the butt end sharply upon the ground. The result may be anticipated, for the gun went off, lodging its contents in the body of John Smith, who stood about three yards from its muzzle.*

No doubt, many landowners of the time, confronted with a seriously injured poacher, would not have been in any hurry to get them a surgeon; thankfully, this time nobler sentiments prevailed.

---

* An irritating know-it-all

I was sent for immediately, and arrived just as the poor fellow was brought home. The contents of the gun had entered about half an inch below the navel, on the right side, and had passed out about two inches above the hip, and three from the vertebral column; the distance from wound to wound was about six inches.

Mr. Daniell was not sure at first whether the shot had passed straight through the body; it was possible, he thought, that it had been deflected by the abdominal muscles and thus avoided the major organs. But on reflection, he ruled out this idea as implausible.

Under the circumstances, I thought it right to give a very unfavourable prognosis, and the family of the poor man were prepared for a fatal issue. The ignited wadding or cartridge passed through the wound unextinguished, and set fire to the shirt, opposite the posterior opening.

Imagine that: He was shot in the stomach, but it was the shirt covering his back that caught fire. The surgeon was not sure what to do but eventually decided that caution was the better part of valor.

There was neither probing nor poking, no endeavours to remove extraneous substances. Nature was left to her own operations, and nature did her business, far better than we, her assistants, could.

Certainly not the way such a wound would be approached today; but in the 1830s, when surgery was basic and infection a constant threat, probably quite sensible.

The wounds progressed properly, portions of garment, and other extraneous matter, passed out at the posterior opening, and about 40 shot passed with them. There still remain under the integuments perhaps 15 or 20 of the shot, but he suffers no inconvenience from them, and is scarcely aware of their existence. The man continues in excellent health.

The surgeon concludes his report with an observation more philosophical than medical.

There is one practical inference which I think may be drawn from this case, and that is, in deep and dangerous injuries, where vital parts may be involved in the mischief, the less we interfere with the processes of nature the better, and I am convinced that much evil is often inflicted by our readiness to anticipate the beautiful workings of the vis medicatrix naturae.

Vis medicatrix naturae is usually translated as "the healing power of nature"—a Latin rendering of a phrase often attributed to Hippocrates, and expressing a sentiment that underlies much of the great Greek physician's doctrine. The idea that the medic should place their faith in the power of the human body to overcome disease and injury, only intervening when absolutely necessary, remained a central tenet of medical thought for centuries. Mr. Daniell clearly thought that some of his colleagues were too ready to perform a heroic operation when watching and waiting was the better option. He may have been right.

SEVERED, REPLACED, REUNITED

Brain injuries were a topic of particular fascination to nineteenth-century medics. In the 1820s, a major debate about the workings of the organ had erupted between two eminent physiologists based in Paris. Franz Joseph Gall believed that functions were highly localized within the brain, so that discrete regions were responsible for sensation, motor functions and even different emotions.* His younger rival Marie-Jean-Pierre Flourens disputed this theory, arguing that his own animal experiments showed that the brain operated as an "indivisible whole." While such research provided some interesting results, it was often cruel—and of questionable utility since nobody knew whether the results were applicable to humans.

Cases of recovery from major trauma to the brain were therefore of great empirical value, as well as being diverting curiosities. By correlating the location of the injured tissue with any mental or physical impairment observed in the patient, physicians hoped to learn more about the function of the brain. In the summer of 1852, *The New Jersey Medical Reporter* printed one particularly striking story, described by its author as "a case of recovery after a portion of the brain had been severed from the cerebral mass, replaced, and apparently reunited."

Severe and Extensive Injury to the Brain followed by Recovery.
By W. MORTIMER BROWN, M. D.

The wound was made by a sharp axe, which, in the hands of a strong and angry man, was driven with such force as to make a

---

* A theory that gave rise to the pseudoscience of phrenology, whose adherents believed that the shape of an individual's skull accurately predicted their character

section of the skull, cutting off a portion of the brain which remained
in its situation in the severed portion of the skull, hanging down on
the shoulder, attached by a strip of integuments to the neck.

Dr. Mortimer Brown gives no details of the events leading up to this crisis, but the phrase "a strong and angry man" hints at fierce passions and operatic drama. To "make a section" is a surgical term meaning to cut or divide: The enraged axman had lopped off a sizable chunk at the top and back of the victim's skull, which remained attached only by the soft tissues. The part of the brain affected was probably the posterior parietal cortex, which deals primarily with movement and spatial awareness.

The man was able, after the injury, to walk some rods with
assistance, and talked in a rational manner by the way. Secur-
ing the occipital artery,* which had been divided, removing
some small fragments of bone, shaving around and thoroughly
cleansing the wound, I restored the flap of integuments, with
the portion of skull and brain, to its proper position, and se-
cured them by stitches, adhesive plaster, and a roller.

It doesn't sound like much, but it was probably the best that could have been done for the patient at this date. There was a grave danger of infection, given the nature of the wound.

The head was kept elevated and cool, a light diet enjoined, and
a solution of sulphate of magnesia, and tartrate of antimony
and potassa, given to move the bowels, reduce the circulation,
and restrain the appetite.

---

* A large blood vessel in the back of the scalp

A mid-nineteenth-century doctor rarely lost an opportunity to get his laxatives out—whether or not the malady had anything to do with the bowels. But maybe they weren't such a bad idea, given the man's subsequent rapid recovery.

The mental faculties remained unimpaired, except for a short time on the second day; the wound healed rapidly, being entirely closed in a week, no unpleasant symptoms afterwards occurred, and on a subsequent examination the severed portion appeared to be firmly united to the cranium, no motion being perceptible on firm pressure, and no inconvenience being felt when galloping on horseback.

I love that last observation: Apparently, the patient was worried that he'd be able to hear bits of his brain rattling around inside his skull during vigorous activity.

There was no evidence in the dressings of the discharge of any portion of the brain, and, in all probability, the severed portions reunited without loss of substance. The case was watched with some interest to mark the development of any peculiar mental phenomena, but nothing occurred worthy of note.

But was brain matter really severed, replaced and reunited, as the author claims? Unlikely. While the body does an extraordinary job of repairing wounds to the skin, muscle and even bone, it cannot regenerate brain tissue damaged or lost by injury—at least, not in any great quantity. It's far more probable that the affected tissue simply died and was reabsorbed. The fact that this took place without the patient suffering any appreciable neurological impairment is pretty unusual—even if the brain didn't glue itself back together, it's still an impressive recovery from an ax to the skull. But I still wish I knew what had aroused the ire of the "strong and angry man" who was wielding it.

GIVE THAT MAN A MEDAL

In 1862, a French army deserter named Jacques Roellinger emigrated (or rather fled) to the United States, where he promptly volunteered to fight in the Civil War. He joined a New York regiment on the Union side, an irregular outfit known as the *Enfants Perdus* ("Lost Children") consisting largely of French soldiers, with a sprinkling of Italians, Spaniards and Portuguese. This motley gathering of nationalities proved so unruly that its commanding officer once threatened to place the entire regiment under arrest for insubordination. The ill-disciplined *Enfants Perdus* were treated with scorn by most of their American comrades, but they played a full part in the war. In the case of Jacques Roellinger, a very full part indeed, as an article published in the *Medical Record* in 1875 makes abundantly clear:

> **REMARKABLE RECOVERY FROM GUN-SHOT, SABRE, BAYONET, AND SHELL WOUNDS.**

On June 29, 1865, Roellinger asked to be released from military service. When he appeared before an army board to make his case for a pension, he told the officers that shortly after joining up, he had been present at the evacuation of Yorktown. His platoon had been ambushed and he had been injured. At the medical officer's request, he showed the panel his scars. The doctor noted that he had been disfigured

(1) by a sabre cut, leaving a long scar, which crossed the quadriceps extensor of the left thigh in its middle third. It appeared to have divided the tendinous and a portion of the muscular structures.

(2) by a sabre thrust, which passed between the bones in the middle third of the right forearm.

Roellinger explained that these wounds had healed fairly quickly, and he was able to resume active service at Williamsburg a few months later. Luck was not with him, however, because he was then

(3) shot in the right thigh, the ball passing through the middle third, just external to the femur.

(4) At the assault on Port Wagner, in Charleston Harbor, July 10th, 1863, he received a sword cut across the spinal muscles covering the lower dorsal vertebrae.

While convalescing from this unfortunate turn of events, he traveled to visit his brother in southwestern Missouri. This "holiday" did not go well: He was captured by guerrillas and tortured "in Indian fashion." Injuries inflicted on him included

(5) Two broad and contracted cicatrices* he declared were the marks left by burning splinters of wood, which were held upon the surface of the right anterior portion of the thorax.

Undaunted, he managed to escape from his captors, and—clearly a glutton for punishment—was reunited with his comrades-in-arms.

---

* Scars

On February 20, 1864, he was present at the Battle of Olustee in Florida. His luck had not improved:

(6) a fragment of an exploding shell passed from without inward beneath the hamstrings of the right thigh, and remained embedded in the ligamentous tissues about the internal condyle* of the femur.

The medical officer examined the joint and could feel the shrapnel fragment still lodged in the soft tissue. Roellinger explained that he had fallen on the battlefield but was left alone by the enemy. Expecting another assault, he managed to pull himself up into a tree using some trailing vines. A renewed attack duly came; he was spotted and shot.

(7) The ball entered between the sixth and seventh ribs on the left side, just beneath the apex of the heart, and issued on the right side, posteriorly, near the angle of the ninth rib, traversing a portion of both lungs. Profuse hemorrhage from the mouth followed, and from the wound also, and, fearing that he must soon faint and fall, he slid down from his elevated position to the ground beneath.

By happy chance, he explained, he had been a professional acrobat before entering the army, which helped him to do so without (further) injury. Seeing the enemy in retreat, he took a few potshots at them in revenge. This was most unwise, for they ran back and bayoneted him through the body. The weapon

(8) passed through the left lobe of the liver, and lacerated the posterior border of the diaphragm!

---

* The knob at the end of the bone, part of the joint

Hoping to finish him off, his assailants then shot him again. The pistol ball

> *(9) entered on the level of the angle of the left lower jaw, through the border of the sterno-cleido-mastoid muscle, and issued at the corresponding point on the other side of the neck. He added that during his convalescence he used to amuse the company by drinking and projecting the fluid in a stream from either side of his neck, by simple muscular effort.*

The medical officer remarked in his notes that even after this terrible experience, the soldier lived "most inexcusably," and

> *at some time, I cannot say whether before or after, acquired the further following embellishments, viz.:*
> *(10) The scar of a sabre thrust passing between radius and ulna, just below left elbow.*
> *(11) A pistol shot, passing diagonally outward and upward through the pectorales major and deltoid of left side; and*
> *(12) a deep cut dividing the commissure of the left thumb and forefinger down to the carpal bones.*

Astonishingly, there were no ill effects from this long list of injuries except a stiff knee. The soldier was granted his request and given an honorable discharge. But what was he intending to do in retirement? Go fishing? Open a bar? Nope:

> *When the catalogue was ended this surgical museum politely apologized for his haste, saying that he was on his way to the steamer, intending to join Garibaldi's army, at that time campaigning in the Valtelline.*

The brave Roellinger was duly awarded his pension. But there's one more twist to this extraordinary tale. It may seem odd that a French army deserter would want to fight for Garibaldi in the mountains of northern Italy, and indeed it soon emerged that he wasn't French, and his name wasn't Roellinger. On the day that he applied for his pension, the man calling himself Roellinger visited another claim office and filed a second application, this time in the name of Frederick Guscetti. He would have got away with this attempted fraud were it not for a chance encounter between the two agents who had dealt with him. The authorities were notified, and "Guscetti" was arrested and sentenced to seven years in the notorious Sing Sing prison.

Except that his name wasn't Guscetti either. It was common practice in some Civil War regiments to assume the identity of a dead comrade, in the hope of landing an extra pension. The *real* Frederick Guscetti had feigned death in a failed attempt to escape a prisoner-of-war camp but was very much alive and working as a civil engineer. The serial imposter was finally unmasked as another Italian, a man called Giusetto, whose greed apparently outweighed his intelligence.

But what of the genuine Jacques Roellinger, the original victim of this elaborate identity theft? He, too, was still alive and now living in Ohio, having deserted his New York regiment after only a few days of service. In fact, the one thing incontestably true about Roellinger/Guscetti/Giusetto's story was his improbable litany of injuries.

A BIT OF A HEADACHE

One of the things that all first-aiders should know is that blades or other penetrating objects should **never** be removed from a stab wound. Extraction should be attempted only by medical professionals in appropriate surroundings, since the foreign object may be acting as a barrier to further blood loss, and removing it may provoke a fatal hemorrhage.

Those with a background in emergency medicine would doubtless wince at the treatment given to a patient in France in 1881— which somehow he survived.

Art. 11814. Singulier cas de suicide. — Un poignard dans le crane produisant une plaie de cerveau sans symptômes. —

On April 8th a man had an argument with his wife on the subject of rent money, which he could not give her. Overwhelmed by her abuse, he wanted to end his life. Taking a small dagger ten centimetres in length, he placed it vertically on the top of his head, and with the help of a hammer drove it up to the hilt.

Not only a strange choice of method but a horribly awkward one to execute.

Having done this he was no better off than before. Not only had it not brought him any money, but it had failed to end his life, and he felt nothing. He still had his intellect, his senses and movement. Deeply embarrassed at having positioned his dagger so badly, he had to call the doctor, who attempted to remove the knife from the skull; but all his efforts were fruitless.

What can have been the feelings of this local practitioner, confronted with a patient who was walking and talking despite ten centimeters of cold steel buried deep in his brain? Sensibly, the local doctor called an eminent hospital physician, Dr. Dubrisay. The two medics together attempted a grotesque tug-of-war, with one of them holding the man's feet and the other the dagger. Then they tried a

different approach by both lifting the dagger by its handle but succeeded only in suspending the patient in midair. At their wits' end,
they took the man—who was still conscious and apparently not in
any discomfort—to a workshop that owned a steam engine:

> He was placed on the ground, seated and held in place, between
> two beams, in the middle of which was a strong pair of iron
> pincers moved by mechanical force. The dagger blade was
> seized and pulled without any sudden jerks and extracted,
> raising the patient slightly, who fell back upon the ground. He
> immediately got up and walked, accompanied M. Dubrisay to
> his carriage and thanked him.

The blade of the dagger was found to be slightly bent, suggesting
that it had passed right through the brain and come into contact
with the inside of the skull on the other side. The doctors were
worried that their patient would develop an infection from the effects of this dirty foreign object:

> Fearing the appearance of the symptoms of meningitis, the
> patient was taken to the St Louis Hospital under the care of
> M. Pean; but he left after eight days, without developing any
> signs of inflammation or of paralysis.

But, one hopes, having learned a valuable lesson.

6

TALL TALES

WHEN *MEDICAL ESSAYS and Observations*, the first English-language medical journal, was founded in 1733, its editor Alexander Monro (primus)* remarked that to write properly on such a technical subject, an author needed four essential qualities: sagacity and knowledge ("to guard against errors and mistakes in the names and natures of things"); accuracy ("to omit no essential circumstance"); and candor ("to conceal nothing material"). To ensure that the articles he published were rigorous and correct, they were first sent to an expert for evaluation—they were peer-reviewed, in fact, just as scientific papers are today.

While most editors had noble aspirations to print nothing but the unvarnished truth, their journals sometimes strayed into the realms of fiction. Until the late nineteenth century, they relied heavily on anecdote rather than hard data, and some physicians would accept a patient's story at face value even if they had not

---

* So called to distinguish him from his son Alexander Monro (secundus) and grandson Alexander Monro (tertius). All three were medics who held the same Edinburgh professorship in succession.

witnessed most of the events at first hand. Unable to distinguish between the impossible and the unlikely, medics sometimes gave both equal weight.

In such circumstances, it is hardly surprising that folk myths and fabrications often made it into print. Take, for example, the story of Mary Riordan, published in a Dublin journal in 1824. Mary was a young woman from rural Ireland who sank into a deep depression after the death of her mother. She began to pay long daily visits to the graveside, and on one occasion was found unconscious after spending a freezing winter night there in the pouring rain. Her health soon began to suffer, and she developed crippling stomach pain that, she claimed, she could relieve only by eating handfuls of chalk. Mary became so ill that on more than one occasion a priest was summoned to give her the last rites. And then, one evening in the spring of 1822, she vomited an object that she described to her doctor, William Pickells, as "a green thing as long and as thick as one of her fingers, which flew. It had wings, a great many feet, and a turned up tail."

Which ought to be enough to ruin anybody's day.

Over the months that followed, insects at various stages of their life cycle were discharged from both Mary's mouth and anus. Dr. Pickells observed:

> *Of the larvae of the beetle, I am sure I considerably underrate when I say that, independently of above a hundred evacuated per anum, not less than seven hundred have been thrown up from the stomach at different times since the commencement of my attendance.*

Mary was suffering from some intractable mental illness, no doubt—possibly Munchausen's syndrome (also known as factitious disorder), which can cause patients to feign the symptoms of a serious, and often exotic, disease. But Dr. Pickells believed every word of Mary's story, concluding that the beetles and their larvae had hatched from eggs she had consumed during the night she spent in the graveyard some eight years earlier. He conceded, however, that he had seen only a few of the creatures himself: Most were destroyed by the patient "from an anxiety to avoid publicity," while others had escaped immediately after being vomited, "running into holes in the floor."

It's a story so outlandish that it seems hard to believe that Dr. Pickells gave it any credence. But it was far from the tallest tale told in a nineteenth-century medical journal—other still more ludicrous yarns were spun in the name of science. Some of these unlikely case histories were doubtless repeated in good faith; others were obvious frauds; but the delicious irony is that a precious few of them may actually have been true.

SLEEPING WITH THE FISHES

One of the overwhelming priorities of medicine in the eighteenth century was the improvement of resuscitation methods. Drowning was a major cause of death, and physicians realized they needed better emergency procedures to treat those who had fallen into rivers, canals and lakes. Humane societies were founded in several European countries to investigate possible new techniques, among them the Society for the Recovery of Persons Apparently Drowned, which opened its doors in London in 1774.* Such institutions brought a new rigor to the study of resuscitation, although there

---

* It still exists today as the Royal Humane Society.

was already a considerable literature on the subject. One example is *A Physical Dissertation on Drowning*, published anonymously in 1746. At the time, it was attributed to an author identified only as "A Physician," now known to be the London doctor Rowland Jackson.*

Jackson's aim was to demonstrate that prolonged immersion in water was not necessarily fatal—and that even an apparently lifeless body hauled out of a river might still be resuscitated, given the right emergency care. To prove his point, he scoured the medical literature for examples of people who had recovered after a long time underwater. Though fascinating, to a modern eye they seem somewhat—OK, completely—implausible.

A PHYSICAL

DISSERTATION

O N

DROWNING

About eighteen years ago, a gardener of Fronningholm, now sixty-five years old, and sufficiently vigorous and robust for a person of that age, made a generous attempt to rescue an unfortunate neighbour who had fallen into the water; but being too foolhardy, he ventured upon the ice, which broke, and let him fall into the river, which at that part was eighteen ells in depth.

---

* Born in Ireland, studied in France, practiced in London and died in Calcutta, Dr. Jackson is a reminder that eighteenth-century medics were often every bit as cosmopolitan as their modern counterparts.

An ell was an old unit of length, equal to 45 inches. It was therefore 67½ feet, or slightly more than 20 meters, to the riverbed—a considerable depth.

He went perpendicularly to the bottom, in which his feet stuck for sixteen hours before he was found. He himself says that he was no sooner underwater than he became rigid, and lost not only the power of motion, but also all his senses, except that of hearing, which was affected by the ringing of some bells at Stockholm.

A strange predicament: stuck in a riverbed, listening to the church bells of Stockholm.

He at first also perceived a kind of bladder before his mouth, which hindered the ingress of the water by that passage though it entered freely into his ears, and produced a dullness of hearing for some time after. This unfortunate man was in vain sought for during sixteen hours, at the end of which time he was taken up by means of a hook fixed in his head, and upon his total recovery said that he was sensible of that particular part of his fate.

A hook in the head is something I would certainly prefer *not* to be aware of. But it's better than being drowned, I suppose.

Whether from the prevailing custom of the country, or the persuasion of particular persons, certain attempts were made in order to restore him to life: for this purpose he was wrapped up in blankets, lest the air entering too precipitately into his lungs should prove fatal to him. In this condition, being gradually warmed by means of sheets, he was rubbed and stimulated till

the motion of his blood, which had been checked for so many
hours, returned. At last he was totally restored by means of cor-
dials, and anti-apoplectic liquors.

The last of these remedies was a medicine produced by Dominican
friars in Rouen, supposedly since the Middle Ages. Physicians all
over Europe swore by their Elixir Anti-Apoplectique, whose recipe
was a closely guarded secret—except that it included a lot of alcohol.

He as yet bears the mark of the hook, and says that he is still sub-
ject to violent headaches. This singular accident, attested by the
oaths of persons who had been eyewitnesses to it, induced the
Queen to give him an annual pension, and he was introduced to
the Prince, in order to give an account of what had befallen him.

Sounds to me as if Her Majesty had been swindled. The Swedes
seem to have specialized in this sort of thing, since Jackson goes on
to give a second example, which at the time was thought so remarkable that the celebrated scholar Tilasius, librarian to the king of
Sweden, signed a declaration swearing that it was true:

There lately was in Dalia, commonly called Wormsland, a
woman of the name of Margaret Larsdotter, who having
the misfortune to be thrice drowned, remained the first time
(she being then young) for three whole days under water, but
the two other times had more speedy relief afforded her. She
died in 1672, in the seventy-fifth year of her age.

If you think three days underwater is stretching credibility a bit,
you ain't seen nothing yet.

*Some time ago, about four leagues from the town of Falung, a
painter fell from a boat into the water in such a manner as to
remain upright with his feet at the bottom. He was in vain
searched for during eight days; at the end of which time, he
appeared alive on the surface of the water.*

So he must have been submerged all that time, right? The local
magistrate and priest were not entirely convinced, so interrogated
him. They asked first whether he had been able to breathe underwater:

To which he answered, he knew nothing of the matter.

Convincing. They next asked

*Whether he had thought upon God and recommended his soul
to him? To which he replied, very often.*

Well, he would say that, wouldn't he?

*Whether he could see and hear? To which he answered, yes, and
said that he would often have laid hold of the hooks employed in
finding him, if he could have moved his arms. He also added
that the fish proved highly offensive and uneasy to him, by the
attacks they made on his eyes; and being asked by what means
he guarded against these attacks, he answered, by moving his
eyelids.*

These can't have been particularly fearsome fish, if fluttering the
odd eyelash was enough to put them off.

When he was asked, whether had been sensible of hunger,
and discharged his excrements? He replied, that he had not.
Being interrogated, whether he had slept? He answered, he
knew nothing of it, but believed he had, because he was some
time deprived of all sensation and reflection; adding, that all
the thoughts he remembered to have passed in his breast, had
only God, and the means of his own deliverance, for their
objects.

A fine show of piety, but what was he *really* doing during the eight
days that he was missing? One suspects that it was something a lot
less holy than offering up watery prayers.

None of these aqueous amateurs could come close to the undisputed underwater endurance champion, however. Rowland Jackson repeats a story first told by the Dutch-German physician Johann Nikolaus Pechlin in his 1676 work *De aeris et alimenti defectu et vita sub aquis meditatio* (*Essay on Life Underwater in the Absence of Air or Food*):

> *The celebrated Mr Burmann assures us that in Boness of Pith-*
> *ovia* he heard a funeral sermon preached upon the death of*
> *one Laurence Jones, a man of seventy years of age, who as the*
> *preacher said, was drowned when sixteen years old; and con-*
> *tinued seven weeks under water, notwithstanding which, he*
> *returned to life, and enjoyed good health.*

Right.

---

* As far as I can establish, the place names Boness (the town) and Pithovia (the parish) appear nowhere but in retellings of this story. They either disappeared or never existed.

However visionary and romantic this accident may appear, in the eyes of those who pretend to have divested their minds of vulgar errors, yet it has met with credit from the most penetrating and sagacious authors who lived at the time in which it happened.

The general point is laudable—don't dismiss things without thinking carefully about them first. But did a teenager really survive seven weeks underwater? I think you can answer that one for yourself.

DEATH OF A 152-YEAR-OLD

William Harvey is deservedly one of the most celebrated physicians who ever lived, despite the fact that he was an indifferent clinician with a notoriously poor bedside manner. His fame stems from the book he published in 1628, *Exercitatio anatomica de motu cordis et sanguinis in animalibus* (*An Anatomical Exercise in the Motion of the Heart and Blood in Animals*). *De motu cordis*, as it is generally known, documents the painstaking years of experimentation that led to his revolutionary discovery of the circulation of the blood.

Harvey's insight laid the foundations for a new era in medicine, so it's hardly surprising that his other writings are much less well known. He also wrote a long treatise on animal reproduction from conception to birth, describing the anatomy of the sexual organs and investigating the development of an embryo chick in an egg. But his *Complete Works* also includes an intriguing and much shorter document, first published in abbreviated form in 1668: a report of a postmortem he conducted on the body of England's oldest man:

THE ANATOMICAL EXAMINATION

OF THE BODY OF

THOMAS PARR,

WHO DIED AT THE AGE OF ONE HUNDRED AND FIFTY-TWO YEARS;

MADE BY

WILLIAM HARVEY,

Thomas Parr, a poor countryman born near Winnington in the county of Salop, died on the 14th of November, in the year of grace 1635, after having lived one hundred and fifty-two years and nine months, and survived nine princes. This poor man, having been visited by the illustrious Earl of Arundel when he chanced to have business in these parts (his lordship being moved to the visit by the fame of a thing so incredible), was brought by him from the country to London; and, having been most kindly treated by the earl both on the journey and during a residence in his own house, was presented as a remarkable sight to his Majesty the King.

Parr was something of a celebrity even before he was presented to Charles I. In the same year John Taylor, the Thames ferryman and self-styled "Water Poet," published a pamphlet entitled *The Old, Old, Very Old Man*, a romanticized verse biography of the supposed centenarian. Alas, the excitement of a royal audience seems to have been too much for the old, old, very old man, for within a few weeks of his presentation at court, Mr. Parr breathed his last. The king commanded Harvey (and several other royal physicians) to examine his mortal remains. This is what he found:

The body was muscular, the chest hairy, and the hair on the forearms still black; the legs, however, were without hair, and smooth. The organs of generation were healthy, the penis neither retracted nor extenuated, nor the scrotum filled with any serous infiltration, as happens so commonly among the decrepit; the testes, too, were sound and large; so that it seemed not improbable that the common report was true, viz, that he did public penance under a conviction for incontinence, after he had passed his hundredth year.

The crime of which old Mr. Parr was convicted had nothing to do with his bladder; this was sexual incontinence, adultery with a woman called Katherine Milton. His "public penance" was described by John Taylor:

For laws satisfaction, 'twas thought meet,
He should be purg'd by standing in a sheet,
Which aged (he) one hundred and five year,
In Alberbury's parish church did wear.

Being made to stand in church in a white sheet was a common punishment for sexual misdemeanors. Mr. Parr was probably required to do so only during services, when all his fellow parishioners could see him.

Having examined the exterior of the old man's body from all angles, it was now time for the medics to look inside it.

The chest was broad and ample; the lungs, nowise fungous,* *adhered, especially on the right side, by fibrous bands to the*

---

* Spongy, abnormal

ribs. Shortly before his death I had observed that the face was livid, and he suffered from difficult breathing and orthopnoea.

Orthopnea is breathlessness that manifests when the patient is lying down, and is relieved by sitting or standing. Harvey's description is strongly suggestive of advanced heart failure.

The intestines were perfectly sound, fleshy, and strong, and so was the stomach: the small intestines presented several constrictions, like rings, and were muscular. Whence it came that, by day or night, observing no rules or regular times for eating, he was ready to discuss any kind of eatable that was at hand; his ordinary diet consisting of sub-rancid cheese, and milk in every form, coarse and hard bread, and small drink, generally sour whey. On this sorry fare, but living in his home, free from care, did this poor man attain to such length of days. He even ate something about midnight shortly before his death.

"Sub-rancid cheese" does not sound like a particularly enjoyable or nutritious diet but is unlikely to have killed him outright.

All the internal parts, in a word, appeared so healthy, that had nothing happened to interfere with the old man's habits of life, he might perhaps have escaped paying the debt due to nature for some little time longer.

Harvey and his eminent colleagues concluded that the old man's death had been the result of his sudden move from the healthy air of Shropshire to the pollution and muck of London, *a city whose grand characteristic is an immense concourse of men and animals, and where ditches abound, and filth and offal lie scattered about, to say nothing of the smoke engendered by the general use of sulphurous coal as fuel, whereby the air is at all times rendered heavy, but much more so in the autumn than at any other season.*

This observation may well have some truth behind it. Harvey adds that the rich fare on offer at the king's table would have been a shock to his humble stomach:

And then for one hitherto used to live on food unvaried in kind, and very simple in its nature, to be set at a table loaded with variety of viands, and tempted not only to eat more than wont, but to partake of strong drink, it must needs fall out that the functions of all the natural organs would become deranged.

The report observes that Parr retained his mental faculties to the end, even at the age of 152; and then comes the devastating conclusion, which I would like to think a beautifully understated piece of professional skepticism:

His memory, however, was greatly impaired, so that he scarcely recollected anything of what had happened to him when he was a young man, nothing of public incidents, or of the kings or nobles who had made a figure, or of the wars or troubles of his earlier life, or of the manners of society, or of the prices of things—in a word, of any of the ordinary incidents which men are wont to retain in their memories.

Funny, that.

Many attempts have been made to corroborate the unlikely chronology of Parr's life. In the nineteenth century, his "last will and testament" was published, containing the recipe of a miracle elixir supposed to have been responsible for his incredible longevity; inevitably, it was a fabrication, a marketing ploy for a quack remedy called Parr's Life Pills. Hard facts have been much more difficult to come by: Apart from one document proving that he was already married by 1588, the outlines of Thomas Parr's biography remain frustratingly elusive.

THE COMBUSTIBLE COUNTESS

Do human beings ever burst into flames? Two hundred years ago, many people believed that they could, especially if the victim was female, elderly and a heavy drinker. Spontaneous human combustion became a fashionable topic in the early nineteenth century, after a number of sensational presumed cases were reported in the popular press. At a period when candles were ubiquitous and clothes often highly flammable, most were probably simple domestic fires in which the unfortunate victim's subcutaneous fat acted as supplementary fuel. Nevertheless, the circumstances in which some were discovered—with the body almost totally incinerated, but nearby objects left untouched—led some to believe that these conflagrations must have another, more mysterious, cause. Numerous theories were put forward to explain the phenomenon: some supernatural, others scientific.

One of the true believers in spontaneous combustion was Charles Dickens, who even killed off Krook, the alcoholic rag dealer in *Bleak House*, by means of a fire that left nothing of the old man except an object looking like a "small charred and broken log of wood." Dickens had read everything he could find on the subject and was convinced that its veracity had been proved. His description of the demise of Krook was based closely on that of an Italian aristocrat, Countess Cornelia di Bandi, who was consumed by a fireball in her bedroom. Her case was reported in 1731 by a clergyman called Giuseppe Bianchini, and subsequently translated by a famous Italian poet and Fellow of the Royal Society, Paolo Rolli:

> XVI. *An Extract, by Mr.* Paul Rolli, *F. R. S. of an* Italian *Treatiſe, written by the Reverend* Joſeph Bianchini, *a Prebend in the City of* Verona ; *upon the Death of the Counteſs* Cornelia Zangári & Bandi, *of* Ceſéna. *To which are ſubjoined Accounts of the Death of* Jo. Hitchell, *who was burned to Death by Lightning*; *and of* Grace Pett *at* Ipſwich, *whoſe Body was conſumed to a Coal.*

The Countess Cornelia Bandi, in the 62nd year of her age, was all day as well as she used to be; but at night was observed, when at supper, dull and heavy. She retired, was put to bed, where she passed three hours and more in familiar discourses with her maid, and in some prayers; at last falling asleep, the door was shut.

The following morning, the maid noticed that her employer had not appeared at the usual time and tried to rouse her by calling through the door. Not receiving any answer, she went outside and opened a window, through which she saw this scene of horror:

Four feet distant from the bed there was a heap of ashes, two legs untouched from the foot to the knee with their stockings on; between them was the lady's head; whose brains, half of the back part of the skull, and the whole chin, were burnt to ashes;

amongst which were found three fingers blackened. All the rest
was ashes, which had this particular quality, that they left in
the hand, when taken up, a greasy and stinking moisture.

Mysteriously, the furniture and linen were virtually untouched by
the conflagration.

The bed received no damage; the blankets and sheets were only
raised on one side, as when a person rises up from it, or goes in;
the whole furniture, as well as the bed, was spread over with
moist and ash-coloured soot, which had penetrated the chest of
drawers, even to foul the linen.

The soot had even coated the surfaces of a neighboring kitchen. A
piece of bread covered in the foul substance was given to several
dogs, all of which refused to eat it. Given that it probably consisted
of the carbonized body fat of their owner, their reluctance to indulge is understandable.

In the room above it was, moreover, taken notice that from the
lower part of the windows trickled down a greasy, loathsome,
yellowish liquor; and thereabout they smelt a stink, without
knowing of what; and saw the soot fly around.

The floor was also covered in a "gluish moisture," which could not
be removed. Naturally, strenuous efforts were made to establish
what had caused the blaze, and several of Italy's best minds were
put to the problem. Monsignor Bianchini (described as "Preben-
dary of Verona") was convinced that the fire had not been started
by the obvious culprits:

Such an effect was not produced by the light of the oil lamp, or of any candles, because common fire, even in a pile, does not consume a body to such a degree; and would have besides spread itself to the goods of the chamber, more combustible than a human body.

Bianchini also considered the possibility that the blaze might have been caused by a thunderbolt but noted that the characteristic signs of such an event, such as scorch marks on the walls and an acrid smell, were absent. What, then, did cause the inferno? The priest came to the conclusion that ignition had actually occurred *inside* the woman's body:

The fire was caused in the entrails of the body by inflamed effluvia of her blood, by juices and fermentations in the stomach, by the many combustible matters which are abundant in living bodies, for the uses of life; and finally by the fiery evaporations which exhale from the settlings of spirit of wine, brandies, and other hot liquors in the tunica villosa* of the stomach, and other adipose or fat membranes.

Bianchini claims that such "fiery evaporations" become more flammable at night, when the body is at rest and the breathing becomes more regular. He also points out that "sparkles" are sometimes visible when certain types of cloth are rubbed against the hair (an effect caused by discharges of static electricity) and suggests that something similar might have ignited the "combustible matters" inside her abdomen.

---

* Inner lining

What wonder is there in the case of our old lady? Her dullness before going to bed was an effect of too much heat concentrated in her breast, which hindered the perspiration through the pores of her body; which is calculated to about 40 ounces per night. Her ashes, found at four feet distance from her bed, are a plain argument that she, by natural instinct, rose up to cool her heat, and perhaps was going to open a window.

Then, however, he lets slip what is probably the genuine cause of the fire:

The old lady was used, when she felt herself indisposed, to bathe all her body with camphorated spirit of wine; and she did it perhaps that very night.

Camphorated spirits (a solution of camphor in alcohol) was often used to treat skin complaints, and as a tonic lotion. The fact that it is also highly flammable is, apparently, quite beside the point.

This is not a circumstance of any moment; for the best opinion is that of the internal heat and fire; which, by having been kindled in the entrails, naturally tended upwards; finding the way easier, and the matter more unctuous and combustible, left the legs untouched. The thighs were too near the origin of the fire, and therefore were also burnt by it; which was certainly increased by the urine and excrements, a very combustible matter, as one may see by its phosphorus.

So it was the "internal heat and fire" that caused the countess's demise. Only an incorrigible skeptic would point out that an old lady who was the habit of bathing in inflammable liquids, before going to bed in a room lit by naked flames, was a walking fire hazard.

HE SLICED HIS PENIS IN TWO

The nineteenth-century French physician Auguste-Marie-Alfred Poulet died before his fortieth birthday, and his name is not associated with any significant breakthrough. But he did write one of the most horrifyingly compelling books in the entire medical canon, the two-volume *Treatise on Foreign Bodies in Surgical Practice*. It's a fantastical collection of inappropriate objects inserted (and lost) in every orifice of the body, including several you didn't even know you had. As well as diligently tracking down the most unusual cases in the literature, Poulet makes some astute observations about them—noticing, for instance, that when patients seek medical attention after sticking something up their urethra, the type of object is often influenced by their occupation:

> *an end of a taper used by a nun, a piece of girdle by a Capuchin monk, a needle by a tailor, a sewing-box by a seamstress, a bone of mutton by a shepherd, a piece of a brush by a painter, a branch of a vine by a vinedresser, a pen-holder by a teacher, a pipe-stem by a smoker, a curling-iron by a washerwoman.*

Shortly after that arresting paragraph, Poulet tells a story so bizarre that I initially assumed it was a spoof, a fake case history concocted by a mischievous colleague. But Poulet is not to blame, since the tale first appeared almost a century earlier in a book by the Parisian surgeon François Chopart, *Traité des Maladies des Voies Urinaires*

(*Treatise on Maladies of the Urinary Tract*). And however ludicrous the story, it came from an impeccable source:

Observation. — Voluntary mutilation.—Foreign body in the bladder.

Gabriel Galien began to masturbate at the age of fifteen years, to such an excess that he practised it eight times a day.

Well, that is a *little* excessive.

Shortly afterwards the ejaculation of semen became rare, and so difficult, that he tired himself for an hour before obtaining it, which threw him into a condition of general convulsions; finally, only a few drops of blood, but no seminal fluid, escaped. He only used the hand to satisfy his dangerous passion until he had reached the age of twenty-six. Being then unable to produce ejaculation by this means, which only brought the penis into a condition of almost constant priapism,* he thought of tickling the urethral canal with a small stick of wood about six inches long. He introduced it to a greater or less distance without covering it with any fatty or mucilaginous substance capable of diminishing the harsh impression which it made upon such a sensitive part.

Mucilaginous means "moist and sticky." The point is that he did not use any lubrication—unwisely, as it turned out.

The occupation of shepherd, which he had adopted, afforded him frequent opportunity of being alone and of easily giving himself up to his passion.

---

* A state of persistent erection

An unusual criterion for choosing a job. "WANTED: Shepherd. No experience necessary. Pleasant working environment, competitive salary and benefits. Would suit enthusiastic masturbator."

At different times he employed a few hours each day in tickling the interior of the urethra with his stick. He made constant use of it for a period of sixteen years, and by this means procured more or less abundant ejaculation. The urethral canal, from the so frequently repeated and long continued friction of this kind, became hard, callous, and absolutely insensible. Galien then found his stick as useless as his hand, and considered himself the most unfortunate of men.

Tormented by "continual erections" and by his "insuperable aversion" to women, Galien became depressed.

In this condition of melancholia, which affected both his physical and mental condition, the shepherd often allowed his flock to stray; he continually busied himself in seeking some new means of self-gratification. After numerous fruitless attempts, he returned with renewed fury to the use of the hand and the stick of wood, but finding that these measures only stimulated his desires, he became desperate, and drew a dull knife from his pocket, with which he incised the glans along the urethral canal.

If this doesn't make you wince, it ought to. The glans, the tip of the penis, has the greatest density of nerve endings in the adult male body.

This incision, which would have caused the most acute pain in another man, only produced in him an agreeable sensation followed by a complete ejaculation.

M. Galien clearly had something very wrong with him.

> *Enchanted with this new discovery, he resolved to make amends*
> *for his enforced abstinence, whenever his fury possessed him.*
> *Pits, bushes, and rocks served him as refuges in which to repeat*
> *or exercise this new measure, which always procured for him*
> *the pleasure and ejaculation which he desired.*

So the shepherd had now started using a *blunt knife* to pleasure
himself. What could possibly go wrong?

> *Having given the utmost possible play to his passion, he finally,*
> *after perhaps a thousand trials, divided the penis into two ex-*
> *actly equal parts from the meatus urinarius to that portion of*
> *the urethra and corpora cavernosa which is found above the*
> *scrotum and near the symphysis pubis.*

The meatus is the opening of the urinary tract, at the tip of the penis. He had managed to cut his penis into two equal parts, from top
to bottom—quite a feat, even if that had been the intended outcome. But surely this would all result in horrendous loss of blood?
Luckily, he had this covered:

> *When profuse haemorrhage occurred, he arrested it by tying a*
> *piece of string around the penis, and he tightened the ligature*
> *sufficiently to stop the flow of blood without interrupting its*
> *course through the corpora cavernosa.*

The corpora cavernosa are the masses of spongy tissue that, when
filled with blood, produce an erection.

Three or four hours later he unloosened the ligature and left the parts to themselves. The various incisions which he made upon the penis did not extinguish his desires. The corpora cavernosa, though divided, often caused an erection and diverged to the right and left. Dr Sernin, surgeon-in-chief at the Hôtel-Dieu of Narbonne, who communicated this case to me,* was a witness of the phenomena of this erection.

Oh my word. Two erections, right and left.

Being unable to use his knife any farther, because the section of the penis extended to the pubis, Galien found himself in new distress. He resumed the use of another piece of wood shorter than the first; he introduced it into the remainder of the urethral canal, and tickled, at will, this portion of the canal and the orifices of the ejaculatory duct, thus producing an emission of semen.

He was now inserting a stick through the stump of his penis for sexual pleasure. Without, apparently, stopping for a moment to ask himself what had gone wrong with his life.

This truly extraordinary masturbator amused himself in this manner for the last ten years of his life, without feeling the slightest uneasiness with regard to the division of his penis.

---

* Dominique Sernin was a professor of obstetrics, chief of surgery for all the hospitals of Narbonne in southern France, and an associate of the national surgical society. He seems unlikely to have made any of this up.

The original French is even better: *"Ce masturbateur vraiment extraordinaire."* It has a certain ring to it, but it's not a phrase I'd like on my gravestone.

> *The long-continued practice which he had in the use of this stick rendered him bold and sometimes careless in its use. June 12, 1774, he introduced it so carelessly that it slipped from his fingers and fell into the bladder.*

Not long afterward, he started to feel the consequences. Symptoms included sharp abdominal pain, difficulty urinating, fever, vomiting and worse.

> *Tormented by these symptoms, he made attempts to rid himself of his cruel enemy. He introduced the handle of a wooden spoon into the rectum more than a hundred times, and forcibly pushed the spoon from behind forward in order to cause the stick to escape the same way that it had entered; but the condition did not yield to the measures which he adopted.*

I think it's fair to say that these "measures" were not terribly sensible ones.

> *He was finally induced to return to the hospital of Narbonne, in which he had been received three times during a space of two and a half months, and which he always left without experiencing any relief, as he would never consent to an examination in order to determine the cause of his disease. What was the surprise of Dr Sernin, when, upon examining the hypogastric region of this unfortunate shepherd, who complained of*

retention of urine, he found two penises, each of which was al-
most as large as a normal penis.

Well, yes, I imagine that he might have been surprised.

This peculiarity attracted the attention of the surgeon, and al-
though the patient at first assured him that this conformation
was congenital, an examination of the parts, of the very ap-
parent scars, and of the callouses along the whole extent of the
division, led him to believe that this was not a natural vice of
structure. Galien then gave the history of his life, and entered
into all the details which we have reported above.

The surgeon used a probe to confirm the presence of a foreign body
in the bladder, and then decided to extract it. This would entail making an incision in the perineum, the surface between the scrotum and
anus—a procedure similar to that for removing a bladder stone.

The patient, tortured by frightful pains, and not experiencing
any relief after taking 100 drops of Sydenham's anodyne solu-
tion, submitted to the operation.

"Sydenham's solution" is laudanum, a tincture of opium in alcohol.
It is named after Sir Thomas Sydenham, the great seventeenth-
century medic who popularized the use of laudanum in the treatment of a variety of conditions. The tincture was a strong opiate
and (usually) effective for pain relief.

The incision having been made, the finger was carried to the
foreign body in order to change its direction, and one end was

turned toward the wound. The stick was extracted with a polypus forceps.

The term *polypus forceps* is still in use today: It's an instrument for removing polyps (abnormal growths affecting a mucous membrane). The patient's symptoms were relieved, but complications soon set in.

Slight haemorrhage, quiet sleep, the urine escaped without difficulty; on the fifth day a cough, which had tortured the patient for a long time, increased. Fever, irregular chills, relaxation of the bowels, gangrene over the left thigh, buttocks and sacrum. All these symptoms gradually yielded to appropriate treatment.

This sounds like the result of infection, in which case he was lucky to survive. Alas, the "truly extraordinary masturbator" did not live for much longer:

The thoracic affection continued, and the unfortunate shepherd died three months after recovery from the operation of perineal section. At the autopsy a considerable collection of greenish pus was found in a sac formed between the pleura and right lung.

This is an empyema, a collection of pus in the space around the lungs. On its own, it's unlikely to have caused his death, but it may have resulted in sepsis, which would quite rapidly prove fatal.

It's easy to dismiss M. Galien as a pervert, but he must surely have been suffering from a psychiatric disorder of some kind. The obsessive pursuit of sexual pleasure is variously known as sex addiction or hypersexual disorder, among other terms—but it's poorly understood and the subject of much disagreement. Evidently, his was a particularly extreme case.

HALF MAN, HALF SNAKE

A niece of the thirteenth-century pope Nicholas III is said to have given birth to a child who was covered in hair and had bears' claws instead of fingers and toes.* Like her uncle, the young woman was a member of the Orsini family—whose name means "little bears" in Italian. The palazzo in which she lived was liberally decorated with pictures of the animal, and she believed that it was her daily exposure to ursine imagery that had caused the strange deformity of her child. Learning of her misfortune, the pope ordered the destruction of all pictures of bears throughout Rome—a measure intended to prevent any further monstrous offspring.

The belief that troubling experiences during pregnancy could have a significant effect on the unborn child is an ancient one, recorded in the medical works of Hippocrates and Galen. Though long dismissed by many as an absurd superstition, the idea gained new traction in the early eighteenth century after the publication in 1714 of Daniel Turner's *De morbis cutaneis*, the first English-language book about dermatology. Turner devoted an entire chapter to the assertion that birth abnormalities were often attributable to the expectant mother's state of mind, giving it this heading:

Of spots and marks of a diverse resemblance, impressed upon the skin of the foetus by the force of the mother's fancy: with

---

* At least according to the sixteenth-century historian Guillaume Paradin, who was not always regarded as a reliable source

some things, premised of the strange and almost incredible power of imagination, more especially in pregnant women.

There was fierce opposition to his theory, but many physicians were convinced that the "power of imagination" posed a danger to the unborn child. A case reported in America in 1837 demonstrates just how long this misconception endured: the story of Robert H. Copeland, the "snake man."

A Physiological Phenomenon, or the Snake man ; Robert H. Copeland.—

This most singular being, perhaps, has not a parallel in medical history. He is now about twenty-nine years old, of ordinary stature and intellect. His deformities and physical peculiarities are owing to a fright his mother received from a large rattlesnake attempting to bite her, about the sixth month of her pregnancy. For several minutes after the snake struck at her, she believed herself bitten just above the ankle, and so powerfully was her mind affected that when she was delivered, the child's will was found to have no control over his right arm and leg; which are smaller than his left extremities.

Despite his deformed leg, young Robert learned to walk, although he always hobbled. But these were not his only peculiarities.

The wrist joint is looser than usual, and his hand stands at an angle with his arm. His front teeth are somewhat pointed and inclined backward like the fangs of a snake. The right side of his face is sensibly affected; his mouth is drawn considerably further on the left side; his right eye squints, has several deep

grooves radiating from it, and has a very singular appearance
much resembling a snake.

Tenuous, you say? But the similarities didn't end there. The young
man's right arm was said to resemble a snake's head and neck. More
disturbingly, it appeared to have a mind of its own, like a sort of
reptilian version of Dr. Strangelove's right hand.

The whole arm will strike at an object with all the venom of a
snake, and precisely in the same manner, sometimes for two or
three, and sometimes for four or five strokes, and then the arm
assumes a vibratory motion, will coil up, and apply itself close
against his body. His face is also excited; the angle of his mouth
is drawn backward, and his eye snaps more or less, in unison
with the strokes of his hand, while his lips are always sepa-
rated, exposing his teeth, which being somewhat pointed like
the fangs of a snake, causes his whole visage to assume a pecu-
liar and snaky aspect.

Not the most scientific language you'll ever read in a medical paper.
I like to imagine the doctor examining Mr. Copeland and then solemnly writing "Appearance: a bit snaky" in his notes. The next
passage is almost a foreshadowing of Sigmund Freud:

The sight of a snake fills him with horror, and an instinctive
feeling of revenge; and he is more excitable during the season of
snakes; and even conversation concerning them excites him,
and his arm appears more anxious to strike than when no such
conversation is going on. This singular being was born in Car-
olina, and moved to Georgia in the year 1829; where he has
since remained, performing such labor as he could with one

hand, and by unremitting exertions has maintained his wife and an increasing family.

When this description of Mr. Copeland was submitted to the *Southern Medical and Surgical Journal* in late 1837, the editor decided to delay publication until he had seen the "human snake" for himself. Alas, the opportunity never arose, so to reassure his readers of its veracity, he appended the names of six physicians, a sheriff and an attorney who would swear that the story was true.

Robert H. Copeland certainly existed: He lived to the age of seventy-nine, fathered thirteen children and worked as a farmer. He also had a deformed and virtually useless right arm—and even if his mother *did* have a bad experience with a rattlesnake during pregnancy, we can be pretty sure that that was not what caused his disability.

THE HUMAN WAXWORK

In February 1846, a gang of Manhattan gravediggers was asked to disinter a body from a burial ground on the corner of Broadway and Twelfth Street. The land the cemetery occupied was being sold off for redevelopment, and all human remains were being exhumed and, if possible, reburied. The gravediggers had already performed this operation dozens of times without alarm, but when they came to dig up one particular grave, things turned very spooky indeed. The experience at least gave them a story to tell their grandchildren—and, more immediately, a local newspaper reporter. As they explained to the man from the New York *True Sun*, the plot in question belonged to a Mrs. Friend:

EXTRAORDINARY CASE OF ADIPOCERE.

Mrs. Friend, it seems, died in February 1830, very suddenly, having retired to rest almost in her usual health, and was lifeless before 3 o'clock the next morning. She was a hale, hearty old lady, 68 years of age, almost unacquainted with disease. It becoming necessary to remove the bodies of those buried in the ground described, the coffin of Mrs. F. was taken up with the rest, and was found to exhibit no indication whatever of decay; being as solid as when first placed in the earth.

As the gravediggers lifted the coffin out of its not-so-final resting place, the lid was accidentally knocked off it. "An astonishing spectacle presented itself," the report continues:

The face and neck of Mrs. Friend exhibited all the fullness which it possessed in life, and indeed, the cheeks were somewhat larger, and, with the exception of the absence of the eyes, there was not the slightest appearance of decay. The surface, however, was covered with a thick, filmy white mould, and upon removing it, the skin presented the fairest, purest surface ever seen on alabaster! The flesh was as solid and hard as the purest sperm, and as perfectly free from disagreeable odor!

You may be relieved to learn that the word *sperm* here has nothing to do with spermatozoa but is short for *spermaceti*, a hard, white waxy substance found in the head of the sperm whale. At this date, it was commonly used in the manufacture of medicines, cosmetics and candles.

On further examination the whole person was found to be in
the same wonderful state of preservation; body and limbs pre-
sented the same hard, undecayed appearance. Of 200 dead
bodies interred in this burial ground this is the only one that
has not returned to dust. The cap on her head, and the ribbons,
had preserved their form and color.

It sounds quite uncanny—but also entirely plausible. In *Hydrio-taphia, Urn Burial* (1658), Sir Thomas Browne's celebrated meditation on death and interment customs, the author describes a body he saw exhumed ten years after its burial: A decade in damp soil had "coagulated large lumps of fat into the consistence of hardest castle-soap."* In 1789, the French chemist Antoine François de Fourcroy made the same observation in bodies dug up from the Cemetière des Innocents in Paris, coining the term *adipocere*—meaning "fatty wax"—to describe it. The phenomenon is rare but most often occurs when a corpse is buried in a moist and oxygen-free environment. In suitable conditions, the combined action of enzymes and anaerobic bacteria slowly converts body fat into a white waxy material that after several years can become hard and shiny. One spectacular example of the phenomenon is a female cadaver disinterred in Philadelphia in 1875: Known as the Soap Lady, she is still on display at the city's Mütter Museum.

As for Mrs. Friend, a few days after she was dug up, her family—presumably rather shocked to see her again, sixteen years after her death—made preparations to rebury her at Harlem, on the other side of Central Park:

---

* Castle or Castile soap, made from olive oil and originally manufactured in Castile in Spain

But, fearing that there might be danger of its removal for scientific or other purposes, they had it taken up and conveyed back to the house, and with the original coffin enclosed in a mahogany case, with a lid entirely of glass, there it now lies, the subject of great interest to numbers who visit it daily.

How tasteful—a real conversation piece, and no doubt the envy of her neighbors. Alas, there is no word on the subsequent fate of Mrs. Friend's mortal remains; maybe she's still propped up in a corner of somebody's front parlor. Still, it might have been worse: According to an 1852 report in *Scientific American*, a large discovery of adipocere at a disused cemetery in Paris was put to ghoulish use . . .

. . . by the soap boilers and tallow chandlers of Paris, for the manufacture of soap and candles. The French are a people of fine sentiment, and they certainly carried the quality to a charming point of reflection in receiving light from candles made out of the bodies of their fathers.

I'm all in favor of recycling, but I think that's taking things a bit far.

THE SLUGS AND THE PORCUPINE

According to an old journalistic adage, the correct answer to any yes/no question posed by a newspaper headline is always no. For example:

"Do these incredible photos prove the Yeti is real?"

"Did solar flares cause the London riots?"

"Has a UFO been spotted crossing the moon?"*

And, most glaringly, "Could *x* offer a cure for cancer?" whether *x* stands for "green tea," "meditation" or "snake oil."†

This dependable rule of thumb, sometimes known as Betteridge's law, applies in spades to the headline attached to an article by the London surgeon David Dickman, published in December 1859:

CAN THE GARDEN SLUG LIVE IN THE HUMAN STOMACH?

To which the correct answer is indeed no. But the case report is well worth reading, if only to marvel at the sheer depths of the author's credulity.

> *Sarah Ann C., aged 12 years, had for the last two months complained of feeling sick at times, particularly after meals. On the 5th of August last, she vomited up a large garden slug, which was alive and very active. On the 6th she brought up two, both alive; and on the night of the 7th she was seized with violent vomiting and relaxation of the bowels, and threw up five more of various sizes, the smallest two inches long, and all alive.*

This is, of course, highly unlikely. The human stomach is a strongly acidic environment, maintained at a pH of between 1.5 and 2 when empty. During meals, when the gastric acid is diluted by food and drink, it can approach neutral (pH 7), but reverts to its usual level after a few hours. While some habitual parasites can survive in such extreme conditions, slugs are not among them.

---

* I made none of these up.

† Or pretty much anything else.

On the morning of the 8th, when I first saw her, vomiting and purging had ceased, and she complained of great pain in the left region of the stomach, and headache. I gave her opiate powders, which relieved her in every way until the afternoon of the 9th, when she felt something crawling up her throat.

Creepy!

This sensation brought on the most violent efforts of vomiting to expel what she felt at the upper part of her throat, and she frequently introduced her fingers to seize what she felt, but did not succeed. I happened to call just when all this suffering was beginning to subside, at which time the sensation was felt lower—about halfway between the mouth and stomach.

A skeptic might remark that this was rather convenient, because it meant that the doctor would not be able to spy the creature by looking down the girl's throat.

As expulsion by vomiting seemed hopeless, it occurred to me that ammonia and camphor might destroy the creature, and that the digestive powers of the stomach would do the rest when the animal was dead. The dose was repeated every four hours for two days, and afterward three times a day for two days more, with entire success. After the first dose of the ammonia and camphor, all sensation of movement ceased; and she now seems as well as ever she was.

Success is here rather loosely defined, since the surgeon had only the girl's word for it that any "crawling" had taken place in the first place. He then offers an explanation for the original symptoms:

During the summer she had gone frequently into the garden and eaten freely of its produce, especially of lettuces, of which she was very fond. It appears to me that a family of very young slugs had been feeding on the lettuces, which the child had swallowed with very little mastication, and the gastric juice not being strong enough to act on them when alive, they fed and grew in their new habitation to their usual dimensions.

So, according to Mr. Dickman's piercing analysis, these hypothetical slugs had survived for days or even weeks inside the girl's stomach.

During the time they must have been in the stomach, she was fonder than ever of vegetables and fruits, and would put aside the meat on her plate, and eat the vegetables only.

Considerately providing her mollusk parasites with their favored diet, a theme on which our gullible medic expands.

The three slugs that came up first were not preserved; but at my request the five others have been kept alive and fed on vegetables, which they preferred being cooked, having at first refused to eat them raw.

What is this, if not proof?

They are now fed on raw vegetables.

A mystifying aside that rather suggests he had decided to keep them as pets. Mr. Dickman concludes his article with further evidence of his willingness to believe any old nonsense.

Another circumstance connected with my interesting patient is, that she was born without the left hand. During pregnancy the mother was frightened by a porcupine that an organ boy had in the street; and an impression ever after remained on her mind that something would not be right with the child's hand.

A scenario that will be familiar from the tale of the "snake man" elsewhere in this chapter. To be fair to Mr. Dickman, many people still believed that the mother's imagination could affect the physical characteristics of the child, but by 1859, most professional medics would have scoffed at the idea. In fact, the story is an unusual combination of two venerable folk traditions, since tales of slugs, snakes, insects and other unlikely creatures living happily inside the human stomach have also been around for centuries. Sometimes known as "bosom serpents," these beasts feature in the folklore of cultures all over the world. Reports of similar infestations were submitted to medical journals with such frequency that in 1865 an American doctor decided to investigate whether it really was possible for slugs to inhabit the human stomach.

Dr. J. C. Dalton, a professor of physiology from New York, made a couple of obvious points that his London colleague had overlooked: Slugs are air-breathing, soft-bodied animals that could not possibly survive inside the human digestive tract without being suffocated and then digested. Not content with mere theorizing, Dr. Dalton turned to experiment, and found—surprise, surprise—that when slugs were immersed in stomach acid, they were dead in a matter of minutes, and completely digested in a couple of hours. The answer to the question "Can the garden slug live in the human stomach?" was an unqualified "NO."

So what was wrong with Sarah Ann? Her illness was probably mental rather than physical—like that of Mary Riordan, the Irish

woman we encountered at the beginning of this chapter, it mani-
fested in symptoms that, while bogus, were so peculiar and exotic
that they could not fail to arouse astonishment and concern. But
whatever it was that ailed her, it certainly wasn't a family of mol-
lusks sitting inside her stomach, munching contentedly on fresh
vegetables.

THE AMPHIBIOUS INFANT

In June 1873, a new periodical entitled *Medical Notes and Queries*
hit the shelves of Britain's bookshops. Written by "a large staff of
eminent medical authorities," it was aimed at the general public,
specifically the "tens of thousands of persons who lack either the
means or the opportunity to call in a medical man at a moment's
notice for every trifling ailment." Both in title and format, it was a
shameless rip-off of the hugely successful *Notes and Queries*, a literary and antiquarian journal* founded twenty-four years earlier:
Readers were encouraged to send their medical questions, which
were then answered by experts.

These "queries" were prefaced by several pages of "notes," brief
and breezy articles dealing with everything from the benefits of cod-
liver oil to the best thing to drink in hot weather.† But in the inaugu-
ral issue of *Medical Notes and Queries* one news item stands out:

AN AMPHIBIOUS INFANT.

---

* Eight months after its launch, *Medical Notes* and *Queries* abruptly changed its name to *The Night Bell*, presumably after receiving a nasty letter from the older publication's lawyers.
† Tea, apparently. That said, "for those who can afford it there is no more refreshing mixture than champagne and soda-water. Lemonade and claret too is an efficacious drink, and really good ginger beer by itself is not to be despised."

A story of an "Amphibious Infant" has found its way into some of the London papers. The subject is introduced thus: "Strange results of very early training: a baby that paddles around under water for twenty-five minutes; a German who has succeeded in making his dog and infant amphibious."

Er, what?

Dr Louis Schultz, of Chicago . . .

I must pause here to point out that "Dr." Schultz was nothing of the sort. Though fascinated by medicine during his youth in Prussia, he had no formal training or qualifications. He was a butcher, and when he enlisted for military service, it was perhaps his skill at jointing carcasses that resulted in his appointment as a surgeon's assistant. That is, until

an unfortunate blunder with the knife, resulting in the death of a wounded soldier, ended his medical career ingloriously.

In short: not a doctor, by any stretch of the imagination. Anyway, "Dr." Schultz

arrived at the conclusion that the reason why amphibious animals have the power of living under water, and terrestrial animals have not, is because in the former the "oval hole in their hearts" remains patent,* whereas in the latter it closes from disuse.

---

* Open

The "oval hole," known as the foramen ovale, is an opening between the left and right atria, the upper two chambers of the heart. This is one of two temporary channels that are a feature of the fetal circulation.* When a fetus is still in the womb, it has no need of its lungs, since the blood is oxygenated by the mother via the placenta. The ductus arteriosus and foramen ovale allow most of the circulation to bypass the lungs during gestation; their job done, they usually close naturally within a few days of birth.

> *If by any means this foramen ovale could be prevented from closing, then he should expect that animals which now live on land only would be able to acquire aquatic habits also; for the blood which passes through the lungs while the animal is on land would be able to circulate from right side to left through the "oval hole" when they were below water.*

If "Dr." Schultz was attempting to take credit for this idea, he was being dishonest. The great eighteenth-century naturalist Georges-Louis Leclerc, Comte de Buffon, had made the same (incorrect) assertion a century earlier. In a chapter of his *Natural History* devoted to aquatic mammals such as seals and walruses, Buffon wrote:

> *By means of this perpetual aperture . . . these animals have the advantage of breathing or not at pleasure.*

Buffon believed that diving mammals were able to stay underwater for long periods because their blood bypassed the lungs while they were immersed, allowing it to circulate even while they held their

---

* The other being the ductus arteriosus

breath. He was completely wrong: The reason they are so good at diving is that the muscles of such animals (unlike those of humans) contain high levels of myoglobin, a protein that stores large amounts of oxygen. Nevertheless, the fake doctor Schultz was convinced:

> *Dr Schultz resolved to experiment. Having some newborn setter puppies, he within an hour after birth immersed them in water heated to blood heat, and kept them under first for two minutes, subsequently for five minutes; and, finding that no unpleasant consequences followed, he soared to the determination of experimenting upon his own infant son.*

Or, to put that another way: Having narrowly failed to drown a litter of puppies, he resolved instead to drown his own son. The *Chicago Times* published a detailed account of this quite astonishing display of parental idiocy:

> ## FISH, FROG, or HUMAN?
>
> **A Baby that Paddles Around under Water for Twenty-Five Minutes.**
>
> **A German who has Succeeded in Making his Dog and Infant Amphibious.**

One rainy, windy night, Louis Schultz, Jr., was ushered into the world. The midwife was dismissed as soon as convenient. The child was, if anything, small and delicate. The exhausted mother was now sleeping; all attendants had gone, when Schultz, pale and agitated, at two a.m. on the morning of September 20th, proceeded to execute his unnatural resolution. Stealthily he took the babe from the bed of the young mother.

That's right: In order to perform this appallingly reckless experiment, he had to kidnap his own newborn son.

Water, heated to about blood heat, was placed in a common tin pail; the reckless father laid his open watch on the table in front of him, and without hesitation immersed his infant with his own hands for the space of four minutes, keeping one hand on the babe's breast, so that the pulsations of the heart could be felt. Schultz stated that it was more than twenty seconds after immersion before the blood found its way again along its old channel, with a bounding percussion which startled him with its power, while it relieved his anxious suspense. Feeling, then, the apparently natural beating of the heart, he had no more anxiety, but upon removing the babe from its dreadful situation, it was ten seconds before the lungs resumed their duties and the circulation proceeded in the natural manner.

As if this weren't already bad enough, it transpires that Schultz continued his investigations without bothering to mention it to his wife.

During the ensuing day this thrilling experiment was repeated no less than five times, the father always seizing the opportunity when the child awoke crying to take him into the other room for the ostensible purpose of wishing to look at and pacify him, but in reality to renew his hazardous experiment.

Unsurprisingly, Mrs. Schultz was not so happy about it when she found out.

It was not until his wife was able to leave her bed that Schultz found it necessary to acquaint her with his proceedings, and he then informed her as delicately as he could, assuring her there was no danger to the child, but a certain fortune to them if she kept the matter a secret. But poor Mrs. Schultz could not understand it, and it is not surprising that the shock occasioned by this unheard-of intelligence prostrated her again for nearly two weeks.

Let's face it, her objections were not exactly unreasonable.

In spite of the severity of the winter, Schultz never neglected the regular immersion of his child five times a day, for periods of time ranging from five minutes to, on one occasion, 25. On this latter occasion considerable maceration was observed, and immersion for so long a time was not repeated.

Maceration is a white pallor, the consequence of prolonged soaking in water. The newspaper's journalist claimed to have witnessed the amphibious child in action:

The boy is a golden, curly-haired, blue-eyed little fellow, and exhibits physical powers uncommon in a child of his age. His flesh is hard, white and shining, and the writer was assured the infant was entirely free from the peevishness and fretfulness common to children of that tender age. A room is fitted up especially for him, containing a large bathtub with a thermometer suspended in it, and the writer was allowed to witness his immersion. The father slated that very often he would voluntarily enter the water, but usually they were obliged to resort to some compulsion.

Further burnishing his credentials as father of the year.

The bath was prepared and the child undressed, when the father dropped his knife into the bath and asked the child to go and get it, at the same time placing him upon the edge of the bath, with his chubby little legs in the water. The child plunged in at once, and appeared to have much better control of his movements in the water than out. He soon handed the knife to his father, although the water was fully three feet deep. Five or six white peppermint lozenges were then tossed in different parts of the bath, in pursuit of which the child eagerly went, and he was fully three minutes under water endeavoring to secure them, as he dropped them again almost as fast as he picked them up.

Spare a thought for the journalist, who must have thought he was in the presence of a maniac.

Mrs. Schultz, although now satisfied there is no danger to be expected from the treatment of her child, is by no means reconciled to it, and expressed the belief that when the affair becomes public her husband will be prosecuted and imprisoned for his unnatural conduct.

She had a point.

Schultz, on the contrary, considers that he is doing humanity a service by initiating a practical and certain method of obviating all danger to human life by drowning, and asserts his belief that the day is not far distant when the acquisition of this

*amphibious faculty will be as prevalent a practice as vaccina-
tion is now, and will be made compulsory, if necessary, by law.*

Strangely, this prediction has yet to come to pass. The editor of
Medical Notes and Queries* plainly thought the whole thing ludicrous, and concluded his response with a withering lesson in basic
physiology.

> *Before the practice of attempting to render children amphibi-
> ous becomes as "common as vaccination", it would be as well if
> those who would essay the feat were informed that the blood, to
> serve its functions, requires to be oxygenated as well as circu-
> lated, and further, that if not oxygenated it will cease to circu-
> late. The oval hole unfortunately provides no means for the
> supply of oxygen to the vital fluid. A still more important fact
> for such experimenters to remember is this: that should the ex-
> periment fail from any cause—and any experiment may fail
> at some time or in some hands—the person to whom the failure
> occurs will be made to compound for his want of success by a
> commitment for manslaughter.*

Mr. Schultz seems to have escaped such a fate, although there's no
further trace of him or his aquatic offspring in the archives. Now,
why might that be? Possibly because they never existed. The 1870s
was the golden age of the newspaper hoax, when writers including
Mark Twain entertained themselves by publishing stories about
made-up massacres, fatal fires at nonexistent theaters and (my

---

* Or rather the editor of *The Medical Times and Gazette*, from which the paragraph was
copied without acknowledgment.

personal favorite) imaginary man-eating trees of Madagascar. In
the absence of any corroborating evidence, I suspect the amphibious infant was an inspired piece of fake news.

THE SEVENTY-YEAR-OLD MOTHER-TO-BE

In 1895, a Mrs. Henry from Donegal in Ireland died at the impressive age of 112. Her surviving relatives included a daughter who
was herself a sprightly 90, but when a careless printer left off a zero,
it was erroneously reported by one newspaper that she was only
nine. As a result of this unfortunate misprint, Mrs. Henry has at-
tained undeserved fame as the woman who gave birth at the age
of 103.

Tales of unusually late pregnancy were a recurring feature of
early medical journals, with sexagenarian, septuagenarian and
even nonagenarian mothers recorded in the literature. Most such
cases were little more than hearsay, with medics happily passing on
a good story whether or not they had witnessed it at first hand. In
an era when it was difficult or impossible to prove a patient's age,
most of these cases would not have stood up to anything like rigorous scrutiny.

In 1881, a French medical journal published an article under
the headline "Late Pregnancy," which at first glance fits squarely
into the same category. But what makes this example so odd is that
it was submitted by physicians at a major Paris hospital and printed
without question—at a period when most medics accepted the ax-
iom that extraordinary claims require extraordinary evidence. The
unusual event was reported by a surgeon identified only as M. Latour; his facetious tone does little to reassure the reader of its veracity.

Grossesse tardive.

We have just admitted to the Clinic of the School of Medicine a seventy-year-old woman in an interesting condition—interesting to the staff, that is. This brave woman lives in Garches.

Today part of the Parisian suburbs, but in the nineteenth century, Garches was a village a few miles west of the capital.

She is known as the widow T. Strongly adhering to the principle that 'wine is the milk of old people' she is an inveterate drinker, and about six months ago, returning home after a rather more prolonged binge than usual, she had sat down by the side of the road, waiting until she felt able to continue on her way.

Truly heroic drinking for a woman of her advanced years.

A young man of twenty-four, who knew her, noticed her in this state, and suggested that he escort her home. The widow T. agreed, and as night was falling and the woods unsafe, she offered her gallant knight a bed for the night. It was not one night that he remained, but four: it seems that his audacity was rewarded and that he had found treasures that were thought to have been lost for a long time. In short, to her great astonishment, the septuagenarian Venus was one day obliged to loosen her belt.

M. Latour's gift for euphemism is certainly impressive. He cannot bring himself to write that the young man seduced the old lady, who later found her abdomen swelling alarmingly.

A midwife whom she went to consult, and then the physician of Garches, summoned in his turn, could only note the fact that autumn (almost winter, in fact) had bestowed the fruits denied by the spring.

This metaphor is at least rather poetic.

To sum up, the beautiful lover is at the Clinic where she is being pampered, or cherished, because the case is a most curious one. The inhabitants of Garches are anxiously awaiting the result; they are even willing, if necessary, to contribute to the cost of baptism and—who knows?—to the wedding expenses. After all, spouses should be properly matched.

This final phrase (*"il faut des époux assortis"* in the original) is tricky to translate, since it's an old French proverb, used as the title of satirical cartoons, novels and at least one play. It's an allusion that would have raised a smile from contemporary readers.

If she gave birth, and it was possible to verify her age, she would be comfortably the oldest mother on record. That is, among those who have conceived naturally: Since the advent of IVF, there have been numerous examples of sexagenarian mothers, and in 2009, an Indian woman gave birth to her first child at the age of seventy.

But did the widow T. have her child? Frustratingly, I can find no further trace of her. It's possible, of course, that she was never pregnant. The doctors may have been wrong, failing to diagnose another condition that mimicked pregnancy. The journal article caused something of a storm in the European medical press—but, mysteriously, things went very quiet thereafter. That silence, I suspect, speaks volumes.

7

HIDDEN DANGERS

T HE WORLD IS a dangerous place, and unexpected threats lurk in the unlikeliest of places. Professional sportspeople seem to have a particular talent for finding them: In 1993, the Chelsea goalkeeper Dave Beasant missed the start of the soccer season after dropping a jar of salad cream on his big toe, while the England cricketer Derek Pringle once injured his back while typing a letter. But these are far from the most exotic dangers to have been recorded by medical writers: Dentures, hat pegs and even hats themselves are a few of the objects implicated in illness and injury in the pages that follow.

Nineteenth-century doctors were particularly adept at finding life-threatening situations pretty much anywhere they looked. Children's games, organized sport, even using a pen: All were thought at one time or another to be hazardous to health. To be fair to the physicians of the past, understanding risk has always been, and remains, one of the most ferociously difficult aspects of medicine. The Victorian cardiologist who noticed that several of his patients were keen cyclists naturally assumed that there was a connection between their heart disease and their newfangled hobby—and in the framework of contemporary medicine, the theory made perfect sense.

Perhaps the most exotic threat to health was identified in the 1830s, when a worrying new disease swept through the ranks of America's priests. Doctors everywhere from California to New Jersey reported that pulpits were falling silent as the nation's clergymen succumbed to a "loss of tone in the vocal organs," causing hoarseness and an inability to speak in public. Many ("a multitude of divines," according to a contemporary report in *The Boston Medical and Surgical Journal*) were said to have resigned their livings after finding themselves no longer capable of addressing their flock or even leading daily worship.

What could have caused this ecclesiastical catastrophe? One sage observer observed that the priests of olden times had preached as much, if not more, than their modern counterparts, and their voices "were the last to fail." So what had changed? Dr. Mauran, a distinguished physician from Providence, Rhode Island, thought he had the answer. The clergymen of yesteryear were all enthusiastic smokers, he pointed out, and were rarely seen without a pipe or cigar in their mouth. Chewing or smoking tobacco, he argued, "kept up a secretion in the neighborhood of the glottis, favorable to the good condition and healthy action of the voice box"—as demonstrated by the habits of another profession:

> *Lawyers speak hours together, and when leisure permits, many of them smoke; and, as a general rule, the leading advocates are very great smokers—and yet, who ever heard of a lawyer who had lost his voice?*

Clerics, on the other hand, had largely forsworn tobacco since the rise of the temperance movement, and were now paying the price.

Dr. Mauran strongly recommended that ministers who wanted to ensure a long and healthy career should resume their cigarettes and pipes without delay. And that is how a major medical journal came to warn its readers about the dangers of *not* smoking.

A SURFEIT OF CUCUMBERS

In 1762, a doctor from Malling in Kent, identifying himself only as "W.P.," sent a highly unusual report to the editors of the *Medical Museum* in London. Malling was a small place in the eighteenth century, so it isn't difficult to identify the author as Dr. William Perfect, son of the local vicar. He was also a prominent Freemason, a journalist and—in his own words—a minor poet.* Perfect developed a reputation as an expert on insanity, publishing books on the subject and eventually opening a small private asylum, a sort of cottage hospital for the mentally ill.

Even before he opened this institution, Dr. Perfect—known as a kind and gentle man—was in the habit of accommodating patients in his family home. Given the exceptional nature of the death he recorded in this article, it is tempting to ask whether mental illness might have played some part: His patient had apparently died as the result of eating a vast number of cucumbers.

> Appearances upon opening the body of a woman, who died the beginning of August 1762, after eating a large quantity of Cucumbers.

---

* His works include "A parody from Hamlet, wrote when indisposed and in doubt about bleeding," which begins: "To bleed, or not to bleed?—That is the question." It is hard to disagree with the literary contemporary who wrote of Perfect that "his verses cannot be said to tower very highly above mediocrity."

It may be necessary to observe that this unhappy woman had all the symptoms of a bilious colic, to the most extreme degree, from the time of her being first attacked to the time of her death, which was three days after her eating the cucumbers.

Dr. Perfect suspected that the woman's condition was caused by an excess of bile in her digestive tract.

In a few hours after she expired I opened the body, and found the stomach dilated and swelled to the size of a child's head, but of a more oblong form, and resembling in figure and tension a large bladder filled with wind: the external or membranous coat of the stomach appeared florid and inflamed; and upon making an incision through that and the subjacent coats, a most amazing quantity of sliced cucumbers, porraceous matter . . .

Porraceous, a decidedly niche word, means "resembling leeks."

. . . and vesicles filled with air, issued out at the opening.

Much of the upper part of the gut was inflamed, and the small intestine was "so much inflated, as to render it impossible for anything to pass through it."

The colon, caecum and rectum were not so much inflamed as the lesser intestines; but, what was very extraordinary, the lower part of the latter was mortified for several inches: the lungs, particularly some part of the left lobe, appeared as if they had been boiled, with several livid spots dispersed over them. The liver, spleen, and uterus were the only viscera which *preserved their natural complexion. The pancreas, pleura, and mediastinum were inflamed; a very large quantity of water was found in the pericardium: the kidneys were inflamed, and the vesica* was in a very flaccid state, without containing any urine. The patient, I was informed, had had frequent motions to urine for some time before her death, but was never capable of making a drop.*

These observations suggest that an excess of cucumber was not the only ailment from which the woman was suffering. In particular, the "water" found in the pericardium (the sac around the heart) was a serious finding with all sorts of possible causes. If enough fluid had accumulated there, it might even have caused the heart to stop beating.

It seems that this is a unique case: Although the recent literature contains reports of cucumber poisoning by bacteria and chemicals, there is no record of anybody else dying from a surfeit of the delicious salad vegetable.

THE PERILS OF BEING A WRITER

In an earlier chapter, we encountered the Swiss physician Samuel Auguste André David Tissot, eighteenth-century Europe's leading expert on the dangers of masturbation. It's a shame that he is chiefly remembered for his work on that subject, *L'Onanisme* (1760), because in other respects, he was an imaginative, humane and sensible clinician. He wrote an influential book about neurology, which contains a rigorous discussion of migraine regarded as a classic even today.

---

* Bladder

Tissot was an early advocate of inoculation against smallpox and opposed some of the more radical measures employed to treat the disease, such as drastic bloodletting. Noted for his campaigns to improve public health among the poorest members of society, his clinic also became a fashionable destination for European aristocrats.

Nine years after the appearance of his famous study of the "solitary vice," Tissot published a book about the perils of another occupation usually performed indoors and in private. *An Essay on Diseases Incident to Literary and Sedentary Persons* (1769) is a catalogue of the various ailments that afflict scholars, writers and all those who spend too much time poring over a book. And the dangers are truly formidable.

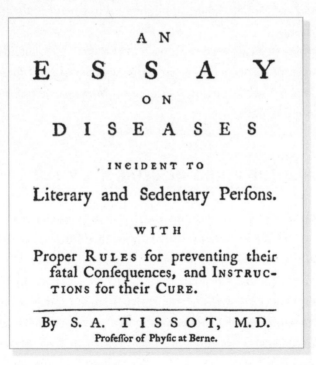

Tissot's thesis is simple:

It has long since been observed, that a close application to study is prejudicial to health.

Much of his case is hard to argue with—particularly when he suggests that a sedentary lifestyle might not be the best way to a long and healthy life.

The diseases to which the learned are particularly exposed arise from two principal causes, the perpetual labours of the mind, and the constant inaction of the body.

Tissot believed that it was not just inactivity that was damaging; overexertion of the brain could also have grievous consequences.

That we may understand the influence the workings of the mind have upon the health of the body, we need only remember in the first place, the fact that, firstly, the brain is in action during the time of thinking. Secondly, that every part of the body which is in action becomes weary; and that if the labour continues for any length of time, the functions of the part are disturbed.

Tissot points out that the brain is connected to the rest of the body by a vast network of nerves, which play a vital role in regulating all our activities. Mental fatigue therefore affects the entire organism.

These evident principles being once established, everyone must be sensible that when the brain is exhausted by the action of the soul, the nerves must of course be injured; in consequence of which, health will be endangered, and the constitution will at length be destroyed without any other apparent cause.

Dr. Tissot was above all a practical physician and, unlike some of his contemporaries, believed that a theoretical argument was worthless unless backed up by empirical evidence. He cites the baleful tale of Monsieur le Chevalier D'Épernay:

> *After an assiduous application for the space of four months, without any previous symptom of disease, his beard, his eyelashes, his eyebrows, and in short all the hair of his head and body fell off.*

Today we would call this idiopathic alopecia: spontaneous hair loss of unknown cause.

> *This phenomenon was certainly brought about by the little bulbs, which are the roots of the hair, being deprived of nourishment.*

The "little bulbs" alluded to are the follicles. Tissot suggests that their sudden starvation might have had three possible causes: an upset stomach; problems with the nerves; or "that kind of low fever men of letters are subject to"—an ailment that apparently throws hair follicles into "a state of consumption and decay."

> *This fever is often produced by the irritation the heart receives from the too earnest application of the mind, in consequence of which its pulsations become more frequent.*

I am (a) a writer and (b) almost completely bald, so on the face of it, M. Tissot's hypothesis is self-evidently true. But far more disturbing were the psychological symptoms displayed by another scholar:

*Gaspar Barloeus, an orator, poet, and physician, was sensible
of these dangers, and often used to warn his friend Hughens of
them; but he was, notwithstanding, regardless of himself, and
weakened his brain so much by excessive study that he thought
his body was made of butter.*

That's right: Reading books (and writing them) not only makes
your hair fall out, it can also create the delusion that your body
has turned into tasty dairy fat. In the case of Barloeus, the afflic-
tion proved terminal, after he became terrified that he would
melt:

*He carefully avoided coming near the fire; till at last, wearied
with continual apprehensions, he threw himself into a well.*

Tissot makes clear that he observed one similar case at first hand: a
medical colleague of great brilliance who many expected to do
great things. But this friend became so obsessed with his work that
he spent all day and night in the library or performing experiments,
with dreadful consequences.

*He first lost his sleep, then was seized with some transitory fits
of lunacy, and at length became quite mad, so that even his life
was preserved with difficulty. I have seen other men of learning
who have begun by being maniacs, and have at length become
complete idiots.*

His next example is a scholar whose name would have been familiar to many of Tissot's original readers—a French priest well known
for his strongly held views and combative manner.

I have been told by a man of veracity that Pierre Jurieu, so famous for his theological disputations, his controversial writings, and his commentary on the Apocalypse, had so far injured his brain, that although his judgment was still preserved in many instances, yet he used to affirm that his frequent colics were caused by the fighting of seven knights shut up in his bowels.

If you think that sounds a bit Monty Python, the next sentence might have been lifted from one of their scripts.

Others have imagined themselves to be lanterns; and some have been known to afflict themselves upon the supposition of their having lost their thighs.

For those just embarking on a literary career and anxious to avoid the (imaginary) loss of their own thighs, Dr. Tissot supplies some very sensible advice:

The relaxation of the mind is the first preservative; without this, all other helps are inefficacious.

After observing that scholarly persons are apt to be in denial about the state of their health, Tissot suggests that friends and family should challenge them to get out of their chair and do some exercise. His description sounds much like the contemporary idea of an intervention, when addicts are openly confronted about the destructive consequences of their addiction.

The only way is to be resolute with them, to force them away from their closets, and oblige them to indulge in recreation and rest, which will remove their disorders and restore their health. Besides, the time they pass out of their closets is not thrown away; they return to their labours with fresh eagerness; and a few moments given up every day to leisure will be amply repaid by the enjoyment of health, which will prolong the course of their studies.

Who could disagree? Exercise, writes Tissot, is

one of the most powerful preservatives and restorers of the health of the learned.

But it's not just physical exertion that helps; being outdoors in the fresh air is important, too.

From the combination of these two salutary powers, we receive refreshment, circulation is carried on with ease, perspiration encouraged, the action of the nerves reanimated, and the limbs are strengthened. Every man who has been confined to his study for some days, feels his head heavy, his eyes inflamed, his lips and mouth dry; he complains of a certain uneasiness about his breast, a slight tension at the pit of his stomach, is more disposed to melancholy than mirth, his sleep is less refreshing, and his limbs are weighty and benumbed. A walk for two or three hours in the country dispels them entirely, and brings back serenity, freshness, and strength.

Never did a doctor write a truer word. And that's all I have to say on the matter; for some reason, I feel an urgent need to go for a run.

WHY CHILDREN SHOULD NEVER WEAR HATS

Most of the articles included in this book were written by doctors, for doctors, and are couched in the professional jargon of medics. But here's a rare example of an eighteenth-century physician writing for children, taken from an engaging but eccentric book published in Germany in 1792. Its author, Bernhard Christoph Faust, was personal physician to Countess Juliane of Hesse-Philippsthal, the aristocratic ruler of a minor principality in Lower Saxony. Faust was a tireless campaigner for public hygiene and did a great deal to promote vaccination against smallpox, but his greatest success was the *Catechism of Health*, a short work that uses the question-and-answer form of the Christian catechism to teach children about their bodies and how to keep them healthy. He was evangelical in his beliefs (some of them rather odd) and was clearly hoping that his book would eventually be used in every school in Germany. He begins with a preface addressed to schoolmasters:

> *This book teaches how man from his infancy ought to live, in order to enjoy a perfect state of health, which, as Sirach* says, is better than gold. You will, therefore, with pleasure, I hope, instruct your dear little pupils in its principles; and as able and experienced men, convinced that the mere learning of the answers by heart can be of no advantage to children, you will have no objection to instruct them after the following method.*

---

* One of the Wisdom books of the Catholic Bible, but not part of the canon in the Jewish or Protestant traditions. Sirach is included in the Apocrypha of the King James Version, which calls it Ecclesiasticus. This is Chapter 30, verse 5: "Health and good estate of body are above all gold, and a strong body above infinite wealth."

The chapter which is chosen for instruction ought first to be read by the master, and then by two children that read perfectly well and distinct; one of them reading the questions, the other the answers regularly and in order to the end of the chapter; the master, understanding thoroughly what has been read, explains its general import.

The master was also expected to quiz the children at regular intervals to test their understanding of what had been learned.

An hour, at least, twice a week, ought to be devoted to such instruction, in order that the whole Catechism of Health may be gone through twice a year, and the minds of the children impressed with the true spirit of its doctrine.

Two hours a week seems optimistic; but Dr. Faust cannot be faulted for his ambition. And it paid off: The book sold eighty thousand copies in the first two years, and was soon translated into several other languages. Faust even sent a copy to George Washington, with an obsequious cover letter recommending its use in the schools of the newly founded United States:

I deemed these books worthy of being laid before you, and through you before the United States of America.

An American edition duly appeared, complete with a foreword by the founding father Benjamin Rush, one of the country's leading physicians. The *Catechism* in fact contains a good deal of sensible advice, and you can see why the architects of the USA might have been attracted to it: It encourages self-reliance, virtue and abstinence—just the sort of values a young nation might want to inculcate in its children. Some of Faust's views are decidedly progressive: He is emphatically in favor of equal education for both sexes, and condemns corsets and other forms of female dress that constrict the internal organs.

That said, Faust obviously had a few hobbyhorses, and sections of the book make amusing reading today. Perhaps the clearest example of his idiosyncratic views is the chapter on clothing:

> VI. *Of Clothes fit to be worn by Children from the beginning of the Third to the End of the Seventh or Eighth Year; or till, in each of the two Jaws, the four weak Milk Teeth in Front are changed for four strong lasting Teeth.*

Q. By what means does man preserve, particularly in his infancy, the genial warmth of his body?

A. By good wholesome food and bodily exercise.

Q. Is it necessary to keep children warm, and protect them against the inclemency of the weather, by many garments?

A. No.

Q. Why so?

A. That the body may grow healthy and strong, and be less liable to disease.

Q. How ought the heads of children to be kept?

A. Clean and cool.

Q. Is it good to cover children's heads with caps and hats to keep them warm?

A. No; it is very bad; the hair is a sufficient protection against cold.

Q. Are those artificial coverings dangerous and hurtful?

A. Yes; children are thereby rendered simple and stupid, breed vermin, become scurfy, full of humours, and troubled with aches in their heads, ears, and teeth.

Q. What kind of caps are, therefore, the most dangerous?

A. The woollen, cotton, and fur caps.

Q. How, then, ought the heads of children to be kept?

A. Boys, as well as girls, ought to remain uncovered, winter or summer, by day and by night.

Lower Saxony has a mild climate and the temperature rarely drops much below freezing in winter; one wonders how the children of colder parts of Europe and the US felt about this advice.

Q. How ought children, male as well as female, to be dressed from the beginning of the third to the end of the seventh or eighth year?

A. Their heads and necks must be free and bare, the body clothed with a wide shirt and frock, with short sleeves; the feet covered only with a pair of socks to be worn in the shoes; the shoes ought to be made without heels, and to fit well.

Q. What benefit will be derived from this kind of dress?

A. The body will become healthier, stronger, taller, and more beautiful; children will learn the best and most graceful *attitudes; and will feel themselves very well and happy in this simple and free garment.*

It was Dr. Faust's passionate belief that a smock was the best form of dress for both boys and girls; but his subsequent campaign to outlaw trousers was sadly unsuccessful. While his views on clothing were often peculiar, there was one aspect of the subject on which he was unambiguously correct:

Stays and stiff jackets are inventions of the most pernicious nature; they disfigure the beautiful and upright shape of a woman, and, instead of rendering her straight, as was formerly supposed, they make her crook-backed; they injure the breasts and bowels; obstruct the breathing and digestion; hurt the breasts and nipples so much that many mothers are prevented by their use from suckling their children; many hence get cancers, and, at last, lose both health and life; they in general destroy health, and render the delivery of women very difficult and dangerous, both to mother and child. It is, therefore, the duty of parents, and especially of mothers, to banish from their houses and families both stays and jackets.

Wise advice; if only those corset-loving Victorian parents had taken note!

KILLED BY HIS FALSE TEETH

William Guest Carpenter was not a famous surgeon, nor a particularly successful one. He spent many years as surgeon to Pentonville, Clerkenwell and Millbank prisons before suffering the humiliation of himself becoming an inmate. He was locked up in 1861 after being unable to pay his debts—bad timing, since legal reforms a few years later would vastly reduce the number of people incarcerated for the offense.

It would be sad if Mr. Carpenter were remembered only for his time as a guest of Her Majesty. Fortunately, an otherwise unremarkable career was distinguished by one case of a truly exceptional nature. Though not attached to any hospital, he was a member of the oldest medical society in London, Guy's Hospital Physical Society, and at one of its meetings in 1842, he told a strange tale about a missing set of dentures:

CASE
OF
FATAL PLEURITIS,
APPARENTLY THE EFFECT OF THE PRESENCE IN THE RIGHT PLEURA
OF A PIECE OF IVORY, CONSISTING OF FOUR ARTIFICIAL TEETH,
WHICH HAD BEEN SWALLOWED THIRTEEN YEARS BEFORE.

Mr H., aged 35, the subject of the present case, was an assistant to Mr Watts, an extensive chemist in the Edgware Road, with whom he had resided for upwards of eight years. Mr H. was afflicted from childhood with asthmatic bronchitis; and it appears that several branches of his family have fallen victims to pleuritic, pulmonic, or tracheal affections.

Broadly speaking, Mr. H. and his relatives suffered from respiratory disorders: those affecting the windpipe, the lungs or the membrane surrounding them.

With the exception of an occasional attack of increased difficulty of breathing, nothing which attracted particular notice seems to have occurred during the early part of his residence with his last employer; although, from the curious facts that were brought to light in the post-mortem examination, I think he must have suffered more or less for some years past; but his high flow of spirits, and his devoted attachment to business, were perhaps the means of diverting his attention from his own state of health. I first became acquainted with him in the early part of last winter. I never found him free from fever: his pulse was always above 100, skin hot, with other symptoms of in-flammatory action.

The patient asked for medicine, but Dr. Carpenter refused. This was a matter of professional courtesy, as it transpired that another physician had already been consulted. Whatever the other medic prescribed was no use, since the symptoms persisted throughout the winter. A few months later, the patient took a turn for the worse:

On Friday the 13th of April I received a note from him request-ing me to call, as he had been attacked with pain in the side and chest, which had that evening become so acute as to render coughing, speaking and breathing almost impossible. I imme-diately visited him. He complained of an acute pain in the right side of the chest shooting up to the clavicle, increased upon deep inspiration: respiration short, and hurried; pulse 140, rather wiry; skin hot and dry; tongue furred at the base and margin, red in the centre; bowels confined; cough trouble-some.

After listening to his chest, the doctor concluded that there was an infection of the right lung: Breathing sounds on that side were inau-dible.

*Considering the case one of active inflammation, I bled him
from the arm to eight ounces, without inducing syncope:* this
relieved him of pain: he could then breathe with more freedom,
and said that bloodletting was always of service to him. I ordered him some calomel, antimony, and compound extract of
colocynth, to be taken at bedtime.*

The trio of drugs prescribed for the unfortunate patient made up a
cocktail of highly unpleasant laxatives. Colocynth, also known as
the bitter cucumber or bitter apple, was particularly nasty, described by one contemporary writer as a "drastic cathartic, exciting
inflammation of the mucous membranes of the intestines, causing
severe griping, vomiting and bloody discharges."

After three days, and despite a variety of treatments and
medicines, there was no improvement in the patient's condition.
Dr. Carpenter sought a second opinion from a colleague. The up-
shot was a new therapeutic regime—the complete opposite of what
had preceded it. Instead of violently emptying his gut, they were
filling it up again:

*An enema of gruel and olive oil to be administered immedi-
ately. Diet to be more generous: some port wine to be given occasionally throughout the day, with good beef-tea.*

A few days later, matters came to a head.

*I had prepared the requisites for administering an enema, to
relieve the abdomen and allow its muscles more freedom of action; and had left him for a few seconds, to get some wine which*

---

* Fainting

he might take as a support through the operation, when I was
summoned up to his room, as he had become very restless. I
went immediately, but only to see him breathe his last.

The following day, Dr. Carpenter and another colleague performed a postmortem. They opened the man's chest to look at the lungs.

As soon as I passed the scalpel into the right pleura, a gush of
very offensive gas escaped. The pleural cavity on this side con-
tained five pints of sero-purulent fluid.

Thin yellow pus, in other words. Just try to imagine what five pints of the stuff would look (and smell) like. Both lungs showed clear signs of disease, but there was one other obvious anomaly, a hole on the surface of the right lung "large enough to admit the tip of my little finger." A little later, Dr. Carpenter discovered what had made it:

After I had completed the examination, I was removing the re-
maining fluid and coagula of blood that had escaped from the
pulmonary vessels to replace the lung, when I came to an irreg-
ular substance, which when examined turned out to be, to our
great astonishment, a piece of ivory worked into four artificial
front teeth, covered with a brownish crust, with a pointed piece
of silver riveted into the upper part of the teeth, which had evi-
dently assisted in fixing them to the upper jaw.

These false teeth were not in the stomach or intestines, but in the chest cavity! How on earth had they got there? The surgeon asked the dead man's father if he knew:

*He immediately exclaimed that his son swallowed them thir-
teen years ago, in a fit of coughing, during his apprenticeship.
I again examined the oesophagus; and we were satisfied that
there was neither a recent wound nor a cicatrix to be found;
and the only opening through which it could have escaped into
the pleura of the right thoracic cavity, where I found it, must
have been the fistulous* one in the corresponding lung.*

The doctor realized that a set of false teeth lodged in the lung was
likely to be intensely painful, so asked whether the patient had
been in serious distress at the time, but apparently not.

*The morning after it happened, he mentioned the circumstance
to Mr Champley, his master, who advised him to take an aperi-
ent,† supposing the teeth had passed into the stomach: it was
thought that the teeth had passed away by the bowels, unnoticed;
and then the circumstance gradually became forgotten.*

Dr. Carpenter surmised that the patient had somehow managed to
inhale the denture, that it had entered the lung and then worked its
way through the wall of the organ before lodging inside the pleura,
the sac around it. He noted that one of the false teeth was still quite
sharp: enough, he thought, to have created the opening he observed. It all seems rather unlikely (you'd expect such a major injury to have caused serious bleeding and altogether more dramatic
symptoms), but it's difficult to explain the case any other way. What

---

* Anomalous
† Laxative

is particularly remarkable about it is that the teeth remained in situ for *thirteen years* before the patient's death.

The report ends with a postscript for the morbidly curious:

> *The teeth are now in the possession of Mr Carpenter, West Street, Finsbury Circus.*

Where I'm sure he received a steady stream of visitors eager to see them.

PEGGED OUT

In 1864, a surgeon from Gloucester, Robert Brudenell Carter, sent a series of case reports for publication in *The Ophthalmic Review*. By his own admission the thirty-six-year-old Carter was "a conspicuously unsuccessful general practitioner in the country," but within a few years, his career had blossomed, providing some justification for the old chestnut that for some, at least, life begins at forty. Carter was an unusually accomplished individual whose achievements went far beyond surgery. He performed with distinction as an army surgeon in the Crimea, and his dispatches from the front were published in *The Times*.

Carter founded ophthalmic hospitals in Nottingham and Gloucester, but eventually became disillusioned with medical life in the provinces. When he decided to move back to London in 1868, it was the newspapers, rather than hospitals, to which he applied for a job. *The Times* made him a staff member, as did *The Lancet*; and the following year, Carter resumed his surgical career at the Royal Eye Hospital in Southwark. For the rest of his life, he pursued this unconventional double life as an eminent surgeon and a prominent member of Fleet Street. At *The Times* he was celebrated as the first journalist to use a typewriter, and for doing so while wearing two pairs of glasses simultaneously.

This unusual case report gives some hint of his literary abilities:

Foreign Body impacted in the Orbit.

G.W., a hale, vigorous old man turned 73 years of age, fell down stairs in the dark, being drunk, some time in the last few days of May. He did not lose consciousness from the fall. He injured the nasal side of the right eye, and bled very freely from the wound; but he did not seek medical aid till June 1st, when he went to Mr Clarke, who found a ragged conjunctival wound and much swelling of the lids, and ordered a simple dressing.

Nothing very remarkable, or so it appeared at first. It seemed that the old man had fallen on a sharp object, which had grazed the surface of his right eyeball and made a small wound between the eye socket and the nose.

The patient presented himself at intervals until the 6th of June, when Mr Clarke discovered the presence of a foreign body in the wound, but deferred its removal until the following day, when he visited the man at his home. He then felt the extremity of a piece of iron, which he seized with forceps and attempted to withdraw. By using considerable force, and after much time, he removed the entire shaft of a cast iron hat-peg, measuring three inches and three-tenths in length, and weighing twenty-five scruples.

An amazing item to find completely hidden in an eye wound. A scruple was a unit of weight used by apothecaries and pharmacists, equal to one twenty-fourth of an ounce. This hat peg was a substantial object, more than eight centimeters long and weighing thirty-two grams.

On further inquiry, Mr Clarke found that this hat-peg had been one of a row, screwed to the wall near the bottom of the staircase; so that the man must have fallen upon the end of the peg, and must have broken it by his momentum after it had become completely buried in his orbit.

I'll be honest, I winced a little at this point.

The base of the hat-peg was still in its place in the row, and presented a recently fractured surface fitting accurately to that of the portion removed from the patient.

Nobody had noticed the broken hat peg—understandable, perhaps. What is more surprising is that the patient had failed to notice three inches of metal inside his eye socket.

When the question arose with regard to the exact period of impaction, no one could answer it. There were the seven days during which the patient had been under medical observation; but he could not remember on what day of the week he fell down, and could only say that it was four or five days before he went to the doctor. Four or five, with an illiterate old man, means simply x; but it may be presumed that the actual period of impaction was between ten and twenty days. The patient recovered without a single unfavourable symptom.

The lucky man. One final question arose: How was it possible for a three-inch metal spike to enter his eye socket without causing blindness, brain injury or death?

Mr Clarke was compelled to use very considerable force to remove the hat-peg, and had to loosen it by lateral movements as well as by direct pulling. Partly from this reason, and partly from his natural astonishment at its bulk and length, he can scarcely be certain of its direction; but he thinks that its point must have been received in the antrum of the opposite side.

The theory that the peg had entered the patient's sinus (antrum) seems reasonable enough, but as Robert Brudenell Carter points out, the possibility that it actually penetrated the brain cannot be ruled out. Forty years later, the surgeons could have taken an X-ray and put the matter beyond doubt; but in 1864, it was still a guessing game.

THE CAST-IRON STOVE PANIC

In the late 1860s, a fashionable new phrase began to proliferate in the medical literature like bacteria in a petri dish: "germ theory." For decades, scientists had been arguing about the means by which diseases were able to spread. In the first half of the nineteenth century, the orthodox view was that epidemics of such illnesses as typhoid and cholera were caused by foul air, known as miasma, which was either emitted by rotting organic matter or generated spontaneously in a badly ventilated or dirty environment. A few mavericks believed that tiny particles, invisible to the naked eye, were in fact responsible—but this "germ theory" did not become respectable until Louis Pasteur's investigation of the process of fermentation in the early 1860s led him ineluctably to the conclusion that it was microorganisms that caused disease.

The phrase "germ theory" was first used in a British medical journal in 1863, but the hypothesis was not generally accepted until long afterward. Many researchers continued to insist that epidemics had other causes—one suggested that particles of dust acted as "rafts" ferrying "atmospheric poisons" between their victims. Other theories were stranger still, such as this one aired in *The Lancet* in 1868:

CAST- IRON STOVES A CAUSE OF DISEASE.

When the attention of the Academy of Sciences of Paris was drawn some time since by M. Carret, one of the physicians of the Hotel Dieu of Chambery, to the possible evil consequences of the use of cast iron stoves, little interest was excited in the matter.

It may not immediately be apparent what possible connection there could be between cast-iron stoves and infectious disease. But Dr. Carret was determined to make one.

M. Carret does not hesitate to assert most positively that cast iron stoves are sources of danger to those who habitually employ them. During an epidemic which recently prevailed in Savoy, but upon which M. Carret does not furnish us with any detailed information, he observed that all the inhabitants who were affected with it made use of cast iron stoves, which had lately been imported into the country, whereas all those who employed other modes of firing, or other sorts of stoves, were left untouched by the disease. An epidemic of typhoid fever, which

broke out some time after at the Lyceum of Chambery, was re-
garded by the same author as being influenced by a large cast
iron stove in the children's dormitory.

This looks at first sight like the classic error of mistaking correlation
for causation. So what's the evidence? Well, Dr. Carret cites the experiments of two of his colleagues, Messieurs Trorst and Deville:

These able investigators have established that iron and cast
iron when heated to a certain degree become pervious to the pas-
sage of gas. They have been enabled to state the quantity of oxide
of carbon which may, as they suppose, transude* from a given
surface of metal, and have shown that the air which surrounds
a stove of cast iron is saturated with hydrogen and oxide of car-
bon. They conclude that cast iron stoves when sufficiently heated
absorb oxygen, and give issue to carbonic acid.

A dubious assertion. It's not clear what the connection between carbonic acid (carbon dioxide) and typhoid might be, but no matter.

General Morin related some comparative experiments which
had been performed by M. Carret, and which, he said, corrob-
orate this theory. Thus, after having remained during one full
hour in a room heated to 40°C by means of a sheet iron stove,
M. Carret perspired abundantly, got a good appetite, but felt
no sickness whatever; he had obtained the same result with an
earthenware stove; but the experiment when performed during
only one-half hour with a cast iron stove, had brought on in-
tense headache and sickness.

---

* Ooze out

But did he go down with typhoid? Dr. Carret remains silent on this matter.

Deville, at the same sitting of the Academy, supported these views with considerable warmth.

Which is hardly surprising, if he'd spent as much time as M. Carret sitting next to a hot stove.

The danger which attended the use of cast iron stoves, he said, was enormous and truly formidable. In his lecture room at the Sorbonne he had placed two electric bells, which were set in motion as soon as hydrogen or oxide of carbon was diffused in the room. Well, during his last lecture the two cast iron stoves had scarcely been lit when the bells began to ring.

And did anybody contract typhoid? This crucial point remains unresolved.

These facts are certainly startling, if we consider the reputation of comparative harmlessness which these articles of domestic use had hitherto enjoyed. In France, particularly, the lodgings of the poorer classes, the barrack rooms of the soldiery, the artists' studios, the classrooms of large schools, etc., are commonly heated by this means.

I cannot be alone in thinking that Dr. Carret had failed to make an absolutely compelling case for a causal relationship between cast-iron stoves and typhoid. Nevertheless, his findings were deemed so alarming that the French Academy of Sciences decided to investigate further, appointing a heavyweight committee headed by the physiologist Claude Bernard, one of the country's greatest scientists, to do so. Its report, which took five years to produce, is marked by Bernard's characteristic rigor. After an exhaustive series of experiments, the committee concluded . . . that cast-iron stoves *were* indeed extremely dangerous—though not for the reasons originally suggested. Bernard found that they emitted hazardous amounts of carbon monoxide, a gas that he had already shown to be highly toxic. It was an important finding that led manufacturers to make significant changes to the design and installation of their stoves.

But did they cause typhoid? The report is almost fifty pages long, but the authors dismiss Dr. Carret's claim in a single sentence:

The facts this doctor cites in support of his opinion do not appear to us sufficiently settled to justify the conclusions that he has drawn.

Which, in the world of science, is about as brutal a putdown as you can imagine.

BROLLY PAINFUL

When I was at school, one of my contemporaries suffered an unfortunate injury. As he was bending over to pick something up, a friend thought it would be amusing to prod him in the bottom with a golf umbrella. The joker sadly misjudged the degree of force used, causing an injury that necessitated a trip to the school doctor. The damaged derrière was diagnosed as an anal fissure, a small tear in the muscular wall of the anus: not serious, but it made sitting down painful for a few days. Somehow this piece of school gossip was picked up by one of the tabloids—presumably after a tip-off from an entrepreneurial student—which printed the story under the headline "BROLLY PAINFUL."*

That was a relatively trivial incident, but I was reminded of it when I came across this rather more serious case recorded in 1873 by an Irish surgeon called H. G. Croly:

INJURY OF THE SPINAL CORD.

A boy named Patrick Donohoe, aged eight, was admitted to the City of Dublin Hospital on the 12th of February, under Mr Croly's care. Three days before admission to hospital the child was playing with the steel rib of an umbrella, one end of which he had put in his mouth. He was on a bed, and fell off it on to the floor. The end of the umbrella rib went deeply in through the back of the pharynx, and the child pulled it out himself.

The rib (one of the metal spikes that stiffens the fabric of the umbrella when in use) had not gone down toward the boy's stomach but punctured the back of his throat.

His mother came home two or three hours afterwards, and found the child with his head resting against the chimney-piece. He had been sick in his stomach, and bled from his mouth and nose. She thought the child had been smoking, and beat him without inquiring into the cause of his illness.

Oh, the injustice! Still, the fact that she immediately suspected him of the crime suggests that he may have been a serial offender.

---

* Yes, I stole it. Deal with it.

She was told, however, by a sister of the boy what had occurred, and on looking into his mouth found a wound in the back of the throat. The child raved that night, and on the following morning, finding that he was not getting better, she brought the child to Mr Croly. She stated that, in addition to the feverish symptoms, the child had double vision. There was a dress of one of the children hanging on a line across the room, and he said he saw two dresses.

It must have been a shock for the poor woman, especially since the first treatment she had offered her child was a thorough flogging. When the surgeon examined young Patrick, he could see an obvious puncture wound at the back of his throat. The boy had also developed a squint and could not cope with bright light. Most worryingly, he could not stand upright without staggering.

Mr Croly concluded from these symptoms that the rib of the umbrella had penetrated to the spinal cord between the first and second cervical vertebrae, and he came to that conclusion from the history of the case and the paralytic symptoms. He had the child's head shaved, leeched him on each side of the spine, and treated him with calomel and James's powder.

Calomel was a strong laxative made from mercury, while James's fever powder, invented in 1746 by the physician Robert James, was a patent medicine with a loyal following. Goodness knows why it was so popular, since its ingredients included the highly toxic element antimony, which provokes vomiting.

There was a difficulty of swallowing. The temperature was taken and it was found that it ran up from 98°F, which it was on the 14th of February, to 102 and 105. He whistled, he screeched, he had the knitted brow, and he threw back his head. These symptoms became very alarming, and he had to be kept in a room with a subdued light. The treatment with mercury and James's powder was persevered in, and ice was applied to the head; all the symptoms had now disappeared, and the child had in fact recovered.

The boy's recovery was as abrupt as it was comprehensive. The surgeon was still unsure what exactly had happened to the boy; hoping to test his hypothesis that his spine had been injured, he took himself to the hospital morgue. There he chose a suitable cadaver and pushed a sharp wire through the back of its throat in the same place where the boy had injured himself:

He found the wire went in between the first and second cervical vertebrae and wounded the spinal cord. The case was, he believed, unique.

Assuming Mr. Croly's analysis was correct, it certainly was unique. Injuries between the first two vertebrae of the neck (known as C1 and C2) are potentially the most serious of all spinal injuries. If the spinal cord is completely severed, the likely outcome is death, or at least complete paralysis (including cessation of breathing). This obviously didn't happen, so the spike can only have grazed the cord at worst. Either way, it's a novel way to fall foul of an umbrella.

A FLAMING NUISANCE

In western Scotland, the name Sir George Beatson is virtually synonymous with cancer care. Glasgow's major cancer hospital, as well as a research institute and medical charity dedicated to the disease, are named in honor of a Victorian surgeon who devised one of the first effective treatments for advanced breast cancer. He deduced that the progress of the disease could be slowed if the patient's ovaries were removed; the operation, known as oophorectomy, remained a standard therapy for over a century.

In 1886, this pioneer of oncology made a startling discovery about the dangers of smoking. Nothing to do with lung cancer—it was not until the 1950s that the link between the two was established beyond doubt. No, the article Beatson submitted to *The British Medical Journal* that February addressed the important subject of exploding belches:

AN UNUSUAL CAUSE OF BURNS OF THE FACE.

I have thought it right to put on record the following case, as it seems to me to be one of some rarity, and to have some importance from a medico-legal point of view. I cannot do better than give the facts in the words of the patient himself, who communicated them to me by letter. He writes as follows:
"A rather strange thing happened to myself about a week ago. For a month or so I was troubled very much with foul eructations."

The polite medical term for belching.

"I had no pain, but the smell of the gas which came from my stomach was disagreeable to myself, and to all who happened to be in the room. About a week ago I got up in the morning, and lighted a match to see the time, and when I put the match near my mouth, to blow it out, my breath caught fire, and gave a loud crack like the report of a pistol. It burnt my lips, and they

are still a little sore. I got a terrible surprise and so did my wife, for the report awakened her."

I don't know what would be more alarming: being woken up by an explosion or seeing your husband belching fire like a dyspeptic dragon. Mr. Beatson concluded that halitosis, normally a mere inconvenience to the sufferer and those around them, could also "become a condition of danger."

> *In the present instance, the gaseous results of the imperfectly digested food had their atoms of carbon and hydrogen so arranged as to give rise to the presence of carburetted hydrogen...*

An antiquated term for methane. The verb *carburet* means "to react or mix with carbon." The carburetor of a car engine is the part that mixes hydrocarbons (i.e., petrol) with air to render them more explosive.

> *... the inflammable and explosive qualities of which came into play when mixed with a due proportion of atmospheric air in presence of the unguarded light of the burning match.*

This is quite plausible, although the explosion may well have involved hydrogen as well as methane. Both gases are generated in relatively large volumes (around two hundred milliliters per day) in the human digestive tract. Most is produced in the large intestine, however, which makes it difficult to explain why it should have exited via the mouth.

Dr. Beatson's short article prompted a rather lively correspondence. A couple of weeks later, a Birmingham physician, Robert Saundby, wrote a scholarly letter that included chemical analyses of the flammable gases belched by other patients. But his thunder was stolen by another Glaswegian, Dr. R. Scott Orr, who shared an anecdote sent to him by an "old gentleman aged about 70, who has since died of apoplexy":

> *"Some five or six years ago I had great acidity and indigestion, and then found relief from Gregory's mixture and bismuth, and, for a good time, found comfort by using these."*

Gregory's powder was a mixture of rhubarb, ginger, and magnesium carbonate, a patent medicine commonly used to treat digestive disorders.

> *"But within the last year or two, indeed longer, I have been much troubled by great flatulency, general puffiness after dinner and during the night, with considerable pain at the pit of the stomach. Not troubled with heartburn or acidity so much, but with eructations of wind or gas, and this of such an offensive smell as to render me most uncomfortable, indeed unhappy, in any one's company or proximity, and latterly the pain so severe, or rather oppressive, as to prevent my sleeping."*

As if it weren't bad enough smelling like a tannery, the poor chap now developed an even more antisocial habit.

> *"About four or five months ago, while lighting my pipe of an evening, it so happened that one of these involuntary eructations took place while the match was at my pipe, and the gas then took fire, and burned my moustache and lips, and frightened me a good deal. It was just such an explosion or puff as would occur on your putting a pinch of gunpowder to a light."*

BOOM, as they say.

> *"My son H. was sitting by me, reading, and immediately looked up in astonishment. He has witnessed the same thing occur either two or three times, and it has occurred in all five or six times. I have tried all sorts of changes of diet, but to no purpose."*

Readers hoping for an explanation of the fire-breathing antics of the two patients were disappointed: The appearance of flammable gas was dismissed as the side effect of an unusual species of indigestion. But four years later, all became clear when Dr. James McNaught recorded another case of the phenomenon. His patient was a twenty-four-year-old factory worker:

> *His work requires him to rise early, and on one occasion after striking a match to see the time, and when holding it near his mouth, an eructation of gas from the stomach took place. To his consternation the gas took fire, burned his face and lips considerably, and set fire to his moustache.*

Dr. McNaught noticed that his patient's abdomen was bloated and unusually taut. Out of curiosity, he passed a tube down into the man's stomach and removed some of the contents for inspection. These consisted of

> *soupy matter smelling exactly like sour yeast, and when it was allowed to stand, a layer of frothy stuff half an inch thick, like dirty yeast, formed on the top. This was full of bubbles of gas which could be seen forming and bursting as it stood in the vessel.*

The gas was flammable, and Dr. McNaught realized that it was produced by fermentation, a process normally confined to the lower part of the gut. His patient had an obstruction in his digestive tract that made it difficult for stomach contents to pass into the small intestine. Confined in the stomach for far longer than usual, they were fermenting and giving off large amounts of hydrogen and methane that could be vented only through the mouth.

The association between flammable belches and gastric obstruction was confirmed by a number of similar cases in the early years of the twentieth century. They include this peach of a party trick, performed by a sufferer who tried to light a cigarette while playing a quiet game of bridge:

> *As he leaned forward he felt an undeniable necessity to belch but, being in the presence of company, he attempted to do this discreetly through his nose; he electrified his associates by producing two fan-shaped flames from his nostrils.*

And what could be more discreet than that?

CYCLING WILL GIVE YOU HEART DISEASE

In September 1894, many of the world's most eminent scientists descended on Budapest for the Eighth International Congress of Hygiene and Demography. It was an enormous gathering: more than seven hundred research papers were presented over the course of nine days, with 2,500 delegates taking part. The Hungarians' hospitality was lavish, so much so that one journal described the whole affair as "a pleasant outing for which scientific work serves mainly as a pretext."

Topics dealt with at the congress ranged from the management of diphtheria outbreaks to the health benefits of cold-water bathing. On Wednesday, September 5, a brief session was devoted to the "hygiene of sport." The Paris doctor E. P. Léon-Petit gave a talk entitled "Women and the Bicycle," addressing himself to the vexed question of whether the newfangled contraption was safe for the poor delicate creatures. The dangers had been exaggerated, he suggested, and the potential health benefits significant, adding that in women with anemia or constipation, he had even found that a bike ride brought some improvement.*

Dr. Léon-Petit was himself an accomplished club cyclist, as was the delegate who spoke after him. But George Herschell, a specialist from London, had an altogether less sunny message to impart:

3. On Cycling as a Cause of Heart Disease.

Cycling, rationally pursued, is one of the most health-giving forms of amusement; but when indulged in to excess, or under improper conditions, one of the most pernicious. I have been led to choose this subject for my paper from the fact that my position on the staff of a special hospital devoted to the treatment of diseases of the heart has given me unusual opportunities of studying the subject. Moreover it is of great interest to me, as I am myself a practical cyclist. I am sorry to say that during the last few years a considerable number of cases of heart disease, undoubtedly caused by cycling, have come under my observation.

But cycling is physical exercise, and the Victorians were all in favor of that. So what's the problem? Dr. Herschell explains:

---

* Despite his rather daringly progressive conclusion, Dr. Léon-Petit was not above a bit of good old-fashioned Victorian sexism. Before sitting down, he opined: "One need only to have witnessed the repulsive spectacle called a women's race to understand what can become of the cyclist who has exceeded her capabilities and thereby exposed herself to accidents."

The chief danger of cycling, or rather the reason why it is more injurious than some other forms of exercise, is the probability when riding alone of being led into an injurious excess of exertion, and the almost certainty of the same thing happening when riding in company, especially with a club.

"Injurious excess of exertion" is a good phrase, and one that I intend to use next time I am feeling too lazy to go out for a run.

In the first place we will take the solitary rider. He is extremely likely to take much more exercise than he is aware of before he recognises the fact that he has done so.

It does not apparently cross Dr. Herschell's mind that the "solitary rider" might be a *she*.

He starts off in the morning for a ride, fresh and vigorous, having previously mapped out his course. It not unfrequently happens that when the time arrives for his midday meal some unforeseen delay may have caused him to have some few miles yet to go. He has perhaps overrated his capacity; or the condition of the roads render travelling at the rate upon which he had based his calculations impossible. But he is hungry, and so he redoubles his efforts to reach the place. When he arrives there he is utterly fagged out and has lost his appetite.

"That cycle ride has left me so exhausted that I could not possibly manage a hearty lunch"—a sentence I have never uttered, nor ever expect to.

Again—the roads are good, the wind is at one's back, and the rider is fresh. The machine runs easily. Having ridden out for half a day or so the rider starts to return. But everything is now reversed. The rider is tired, and the wind is against him. Moreover he has been led by the easiness of the outward journey to go much further than he had intended; so that by the time he reaches home he is in the vernacular of the cyclist 'baked'.

In 1890s cycling slang, *baked* meant "extremely tired" rather than the modern surfer-dude sense of "intoxicated by drugs." That said, given recent scandals in the world of cycling, perhaps the latter isn't so far off the mark.

The commonest way however in which the cyclist does himself harm is in climbing hills. He is nearing the top of the hill, the heart is dilated with the strain put upon it by the increased arterial tension. If the rider were now to stop to recover himself no harm would be done. But in too many cases he does not do so. Only a few more revolutions of the wheel will be required to carry him to the top. So he redoubles his exertions, and puts further strain upon a heart already taxed to the utmost limit of its capacity. But in those few moments, damage has been done to the heart from which it perhaps cannot recover.

Dr. Herschell adds that his concern is mainly for recreational cyclists rather than serious road racers. But the experts are not exempt from such danger, since they are "deliberately sacrificing their future health for the sake of winning a few prizes."

Another very wicked thing is what is known as a "hill-climbing contest". If people were to deliberately set themselves to devise a method of riding which should be as injurious as possible they could not hit upon a better one. Hills of the steepest gradient are deliberately selected, and the competitors ride up them against time. Nothing more suicidal, or more certain to produce heart disease, can possibly be imagined.

What on earth would he have made of the Tour de France, with its regular ascents of mountain peaks? On a single day of the 2017 Tour (Stage 9), competitors rode 180 kilometers through the Jura Mountains, during which they climbed 4,600 meters. In climbing the Grand Colombier, exactly halfway through the stage, they had to propel themselves up an eye-watering gradient of 22 percent for over 3 kilometers.

Dr. Herschell then lists a number of precautions that he suggests the leisure cyclist should take "to prevent this fascinating sport from injuring us":

1. *The use of a low gear.*
2. *The upright position in riding. The stooping posture so affected by the modern cyclist, by contracting the chest, prevents the proper expansion of the lungs, and by interfering with the aeration of the blood, causes the condition of breathlessness to come on quicker.*
3. *Adequate food when riding, and the avoidance of muscle poisons such as beef-tea.*
4. *The cyclist must avoid the advertised preparations of kola and coca. These by numbing the sense of weariness, enable*

injuriously excessive work to be done, almost without the knowledge of the rider.

Kola nut contains caffeine and is relatively innocuous, but coca leaves are used to make cocaine, the consumption of which is generally frowned upon in competitive sport.*

5. *On no account should the cyclist continue riding after he has commenced to feel short of breath, or when there is the slightest sensation of uneasiness in the chest.*

Duly noted. Any club cyclists who followed Dr. Herschell's advice to the letter would have been denying themselves much of the benefit they could otherwise expect from their hobby. Raising the heart rate, and getting out of breath, is the whole point of aerobic exercise: It helps to strengthen the heart muscle and improve the circulation and (within reason) is unambiguously a Good Thing. These days, cycling is even recommended to some patients in chronic heart failure to improve their cardiac function.

Despite his position at a specialist heart hospital, Dr. Herschell published very little on cardiac disease. He was highly regarded as an expert on disorders of the digestive tract, and his textbook on the subject ran to several editions. He thoughtfully included a short chapter of recipes for those with delicate stomachs, and a few years after his death, these were excerpted and published as a slim volume called *Cookery for Dyspeptics*. I don't know if any recipe book has ever had a better title, but somehow I doubt it.

---

* The most celebrated "preparation of kola and coca" was Coca-Cola, which first went on sale in 1886. However, the drink was barely known in Europe until a bottling plant opened in France in 1919, so Dr. Herschell was probably unaware of its existence.

Sources

INTRODUCTION

"Sudden protrusion of the whole of the intestines into the scrotum," *London Medical Gazette* 3, no. 72 (1829), 654.

James Young Simpson, "General observations on the Roman medicine-stamps found in Great Britain," *Monthly Journal of Medical Science* 12, no. 16 (1851), 338–354.

1. UNFORTUNATE PREDICAMENTS

A FORK UP THE ANUS

Robert Payne, "An account of a fork put up the anus, that was afterwards drawn out through the buttock; communicated in a letter to the publisher, by Mr. Robert Payne, Surgeon at Lowestofft," *Philosophical Transactions* 33, no. 391 (1724), 408–409.

SWALLOWING KNIVES IS BAD FOR YOU

Alexander Marcet, "Account of a man who lived ten years after having swallowed a number of clasp-knives; with a description of the appearances of the body after death," *Medico-Chirurgical Transactions* 12, pt. 1 (1823), 52–63.

THE GOLDEN PADLOCK

"Case of infibulation, followed by a schirrous affection of the prepuce," *London Medical and Physical Journal* 58, no. 345 (1827), 558–559.

THE BOY WHO GOT HIS WICK STUCK IN A CANDLESTICK

M. Marx, "Chirurgie clinique de l'Hôtel-Dieu," *Répertoire Général d'Anatomie et de Physiologie Pathologiques, et de Clinique Chirurgicale* 3 (1827), 108–109.

SHOT BY A TOASTING FORK

Thomas Davis, "Singular case of a foreign body found in the heart of a boy," *Transactions of the Provincial Medical and Surgical Association* 2 (1834), 357–360.

MR. DENDY'S EGGCUP CASE

Walter Dendy, "Discovery of a large egg-cup in the ileum of a man," *Lancet* 21, no. 543 (1834), 675–677.

BROKEN GLASS AND BOILED CABBAGE

Thomas Mitchell, *Materia Medica and Therapeutics* (Philadelphia: J. B. Lippincott, 1857), 343.

Antoine Portal, *Observations sur les Effets des Vapeurs Méphitiques dans L'Homme, sur les Noyés, sur les Enfans qui Paroissent Morts en Naissant et sur la Rage* (Paris: Imprimerie Royale, 1787), 410–411; translated in "Swallowing pins and needles," *London Medical Gazette* 23, no. 586 (1839), 799–800.

HONKING LIKE A GOOSE

K. Burow, "On the removal of the larynx of a goose from that of a child by tracheotomy," *British and Foreign Medico-Chirurgical Review* 9 (1850), 260–261.

PENIS IN A BOTTLE

A. B. Shipman, "Novel effects of potassium—foreign bodies in the urethra—catalepsy," *Boston Medical and Surgical Journal* 41, no. 2 (1849), 33–37.

THE COLONIC CARPENTRY KIT

Andrew Valentine Kirwan, *The Ports, Arsenals, and Dockyards of France* (London: James Fraser, 1841), 138.

"Foreign body in the colon transversum," *Medical Times and Gazette* 2, no. 596 (1861), 564.

SUFFOCATED BY A FISH

Kajari Roy, Pankaj Kundra and M. Ravishankar, "Unusual foreign body airway
obstruction after laryngeal mask airway insertion," *Anesthesia and Analgesia*
101, no. 1 (2005), 294–295.

"Extraordinary death," *British Medical Journal* 1, no. 119 (1863), 369.

Norman Chevers, *A Manual of Medical Jurisprudence for India* (Calcutta:
Thacker, Vining & Co., 1870), 619.

Syed Rizwan Ali and Atul C. Mehta, "Alive in the airways: live endobronchial
foreign bodies," *Chest* 151, no. 2 (2017), 481–491.

2. MYSTERIOUS ILLNESSES

A HIDEOUS THING HAPPENED IN HIGH HOLBORN

Benjamin Ward Richardson, "Vacation lectures on fibrinous deposition in the
heart," *British Medical Journal* 1, no. 161 (1860), 65–68.

Edward May, *A most certaine and true Relation of a strange Monster or Serpent,
found in the left Ventricle of the Heart of John Pennant, Gentleman, of the Age of
21 Yeares* (London: Printed by George Miller, 1639).

THE INCREDIBLE SLEEPING WOMAN

Terence Brady, "An account of an extraordinary sleepy woman, near Mons, in
Hainault," *Medical Observations and Inquiries* 1 (1757), 280–285.

THE DREADFUL MORTIFICATION

Charlton Wollaston, "Extract of a letter from Charlton Wollaston, M.D. F.R.S. to
William Heberden, M.D. F.R.S. dated Bury St Edmund's April 13, 1762,
relating to the case of mortification of limbs in a family at Wattisham in
Suffolk," *Philosophical Transactions* 52 (1761), 523–526.

THE HUMAN PINCUSHION

"The Copenhagen needle patient," *Medico-Chirurgical Review* 7, no 22 (1825),
559–562.

THE MAN WHO FOUGHT A DUEL IN HIS SLEEP

"A singular case of somnambulism," *London Medical Repository* 6 (1816), 475–478.

THE MYSTERY OF THE EXPLODING TEETH

W. H. Atkinson, "Explosion of teeth with audible report," *Dental Cosmos* 2, no. 6 (1861), 318–319.

J. Phelps Hibler, *Pathology and Therapeutics of Dentistry* (St. Louis: James Hogan, 1874), 28.

THE WOMAN WHO PEED THROUGH HER NOSE

S. A. Arnold, "Case of paruria erratica, or uroplania," *New England Journal of Medicine and Surgery* 14, no. 4 (1825), 337–358.

THE BOY WHO VOMITED HIS OWN TWIN

"A foetus vomited by a boy," *London Medical and Surgical Journal* 6, no. 151 (1835), 663.

"Foetus monstrueux de Syra," *Comptes Rendus Hebdomadaires des Séances de l'Académie des Sciences* 3 (1836), 52–53.

R. Yaacob et al., "The entrapped twin: a case of fetus-in-fetu," *BMJ Case Reports* (2017), doi:10.1136/bcr-2017-220801.

THE CASE OF THE LUMINOUS PATIENTS

Sir Henry Marsh, "On the evolution of light from the living human subject," *Provincial Medical Journal* 2, no. 9 (1842), 163–172.

Robert Boyle, Peter Shaw (ed.), *The Philosophical Works of the Honourable Robert Boyle Esq* (3 vols; London: Innys & Manby & Longman, 1738), 3: 168–169.

THE MISSING PEN

"An extraordinary injury," *Chicago Medical Journal and Examiner* 56, no. 3 (1888), 182–183.

3. DUBIOUS REMEDIES

Polydore Vergil (trans. Thomas Langley), *The Works of the Famous Antiquary, Polidore Virgil, Containing the Original of all Arts, Sciences, Mysteries, Orders, Rites, and Ceremonies, both Ecclesiastical and Civil: a Work Useful for all Divines, Historians, Lawyers, and all Artificers* (London: printed for Simon Miller, 1663), 59.

David Ramsey, *An Eulogium upon Benjamin Rush, M.D., Professor of the Institutes and Practice of Medicine and of Clinical Practice in the University of Pennsylvania* (Philadelphia: Bradford & Inskeep, 1813), 39.

Nicholas Culpeper, *Pharmacopoeia Londinensis, or, the London Dispensatory* (London: Sawbridge, 1683), 76–77.

DEATH OF AN EARL

Kenneth Dewhurst, "Some letters of Dr. Charles Goodall (1642–1712) to Locke, Slone, and Sir Thomas Millington," *Journal of the History of Medicine and Allied Sciences* 17, no. 4 (1962), 487–508.
"Anecdota Bodleiana: Unpublished Fragments from the Bodleian," *Provincial Medical and Surgical Journal* 10, no. 5 (1846), 54–55.

THE TOBACCO-SMOKE ENEMA

Samuel Auguste David Tissot (ed. John Wesley), *Advices, with Respect to Health. Extracted from a Late Author* (Bristol: W. Pine, 1769), 150–153.

SALIVA AND CROW'S VOMIT

V. L. Brera, "On the exhibition of remedies externally by frictions with saliva," *Annals of Medicine* 3 (1799), 190–193.
Salvatore de Renzi, *Storia della Medicina Italiana* (5 vols; Naples: Filiatre-Sebezio, 1847) 5: 654–655.

THE PIGEON'S-RUMP CURE

Carl Canstatt, *Handbuch der medicinischen Klinik* (5 vols; Erlangen: Ferdinand Enke, 1843), 3: 390.
"Ein sonderbares Mittel gegen die Eklampsie der Kinder," *Journal für Kinderkrankheiten* 16, nos. 1-2 (1851), 159–160.
J. F. Weisse, "Ein Beitrag zu Dr. Blik's Mittheilung über Taubensteisskur gegen Eklampsie der Kinder," *Journal für Kinderkrankheiten* 16, nos. 3-4 (1851), 381–383.
"Review XII," *British and Foreign Medico-Chirurgical Review* 22 (1858), 112–128.

MERCURY CIGARETTES

"Digest of the journals," *London Journal of Medicine* 3, no. 33 (1851), 840–849.
W. E. Bowman, "Medicated cigarettes," *Canada Lancet* 1, no. 3 (1863), 19.

THE TAPEWORM TRAP

"Editorial correspondence," *Medical and Surgical Reporter* 9, no. 9 (1856), 430–433.
Alpheus Myers, "Tape-worm Trap," US Patent no. 11942, 1854.

A. G. Wilkinson, "The tape-worm, and kousso as an anthelmintic," *Medical and Surgical Reporter* 8, no 4 (1862), 82–86.

THE PORT-WINE ENEMA

H. Llewellyn Williams, "Port wine enemata as a substitute for transfusion of blood in cases of post partum haemorrhage," *British Medical Journal* 1, no. 88 (1858), 739.

THE SNAKE-DUNG SALESMAN

John Hastings, *An Inquiry into the Medicinal Value of the Excreta of Reptiles* (London: Longman, 1862).
"Reviews and notices," *British Medical Journal* 1, no. 63 (1862), 284–286.
"Reviews and notices of books," *Lancet* 79, no. 2012 (1862), 305–307.
"Court of Queen's Bench: Ex parte Hastings," *Justice of the Peace* 26, no. 20 (1862), 310.

4. HORRIFYING OPERATIONS

Tobias Smollett, *The Adventures of Roderick Random* (Oxford: Oxford University Press, 2008), 86.
Lorenz Heister, *A General System of Surgery in Three Parts* (London: printed for W. Innys, 1750), 24.

THE CASE OF THE DRUNKEN DUTCHMAN'S GUTS

William Bray (ed.), *The Diary and Correspondence of John Evelyn, FRS* (4 vols; London: Bell and Daldy, 1870), 1: 29–30.
Daniel Lakin, *A Miraculous Cure of the Prusian Swallow-Knife* (London: I. Okes, 1642).
Thomas Barnes, "Account of William Dempster, who swallowed a table-knife nine inches long; with a notice of a similar case in a Prussian knife-eater," *Edinburgh Philosophical Journal* 11, no. 22 (1824), 319–326.
William Oliver, "A letter from Dr. William Oliver to the publisher, giving his remarks in a late journey into Denmark and Holland," *Philosophical Transactions* 23 (1703), 1400–1410.

IF YOU CAN'T FIND A SURGEON . . .

Rev. Dean Copping, FRS, "Extracts of two letters from the Revd Dean Copping, FRS to the President, concerning the caesarian operation performed by an ignorant butcher; and concerning the extraordinary skeleton mentioned in the foregoing article," *Philosophical Transactions* 41 (1740), 814–819.

THE SELF-INFLICTED LITHOTRIPSY

V. Rogozov and N. Bermel, "Auto-appendectomy in the Antarctic: case report," *BMJ* 339 (2009), b4965.

Rosie Llewellyn-Jones, "Martin, Claude," *Oxford Dictionary of National Biography*, https://doi.org/10.1093/ref:odnb/63526.

Samuel Charles Hill, *The Life of Claud Martin, Major-General in the Army of the Honourable East India Company* (Calcutta: Thacker, Spink & Co., 1901), 147.

"Col. Martin on destroying the stone in the bladder," *Medical and Physical Journal* 1, no. 2 (1799), 120–124.

A HIGH PAIN THRESHOLD

Dickinson Crompton, "Reminiscences of provincial surgery under somewhat exceptional circumstances," *Guy's Hospital Reports* 44 (1887), 137–166.

A WINDOW IN HIS CHEST

Chevalier Richerand, "Case of excision of a portion of the ribs, and also of the pleura," *Medico-Chirurgical Journal* 1, no. 2 (1818), 184–186.

"Histoire d'une résection des côtes et de la pléure," *Edinburgh Medical and Surgical Journal* 14, no. 57 (1818), 647–652.

THE SAD CASE OF HOO LOO

"The Chinese peasant Hoo Loo: his removal to England; operation performed on him at Guy's Hospital; remarks on the operation by Mr. W. Simpson, and by J. M. Titley, M.D.," *Chinese Repository* 3, no. 11 (1835), 489–496.

"Guy's Hospital," *Lancet* 16, no. 398 (1831), 86–89.

W. Simpson, "The operation on Hoo Loo," *Lancet* 16, no. 399 (1831), 110–111.

ALL AT SEA

Alexander Starbuck, *History of the American Whale Fishery from its Earliest Inception to the Year 1876* (Washington, DC: Government Printing Office, 1878), 466.

"Extraordinary operation on the subclavian vein, by a ship's mate; recovery," *Scalpel* 6, no 21 (1853), 311–313.

AN EXTRAORDINARY SURGICAL OPERATION

"Extraordinary surgical operation," *Medical and Surgical Reporter* 11, no. 1
(1858), 25–28.

"Editor's table," *San Francisco Medical Press* 3, no. 12 (1862), 226–243.

5. REMARKABLE RECOVERIES

William Maiden, *An Account of a Case of Recovery after an Extraordinary Accident,
by Which the Shaft of a Chaise Had Been Forced through the Thorax* (London:
T. Bayley, 1812).

THE WANDERING MUSKET BALL

Robert Fielding, "A brief narrative of the shot of Dr. Robert Fielding with a
musket-bullet, and its strange manner of coming out of his head, where it had
lain near thirty years. Written by himself," *Philosophical Transactions* 26, no.
320 (1708), 317–319.

THE MILLER'S TALE

John Belchier, "An account of the man whose arm with the shoulder-blade was torn
off by a mill, the 15th of August 1737," *Philosophical Transactions* 40, no. 449
(1738), 313–316.

IN ONE SIDE AND OUT THE OTHER

Henry Yates Carter, "Case of a gun-shot wound of the head," *Medical Facts and
Observations* 6 (1795), 91–95.

A BAYONET THROUGH THE HEAD

Jean Baptiste Barthélemy, *Notice Biographique du Docteur Urbain Fardeau* (Paris:
Édouard Bautruche, 1846).

Urbain-Jean Fardeau, "Observation sur une plaie de tête faite par une bayonette
lancée par un boulet," *Journal Général de Médecine, de Chirugie et de
Pharmacie* 35 (1809), 287–291.

AN INTERESTING AND REMARKABLE ACCIDENT

[Editorial], *Medical News* 49 (1886), 600.

Roswell Park, "Fracture of the atlas: separation of a fragment and its subsequent
extrusion through the mouth," *Buffalo Medical Journal* 68, no. 6 (1913),
312–313.

Eugene Mindell, "James Platt White, MD (1811–1881): his interesting and remarkable accident," *Clinical Orthopaedics and Related Research* 430 (2005), 227–231.

THE LUCKY PRUSSIAN

J. M. Chelius (trans. J. F. South), *A System of Surgery* (3 vols.; Philadelphia: Lea & Blanchard, 1847), 1: 485–487.

George Guthrie, *On Wounds and Injuries of the Chest* (London: Henry Renshaw and John Churchill, 1848), 103.

A CASE FOR DR. COFFIN

E. Q. Sewell, "Lateral transfixture of the chest by a scythe blade, followed by complete recovery, with remarks," *British American Journal of Medical and Physical Science* 4, no. 10 (1849), 270–272.

THE HEALING POWER OF NATURE

Edward Daniell, "Extraordinary case of gun-shot wound, where the charge passed from the navel to the back, without fatal consequences," *Provincial Medical and Surgical Journal* 8, no. 24 (1844), 367–368.

SEVERED, REPLACED, REUNITED

W. Mortimer Brown, "Severe and extensive injury to the brain followed by recovery," *New Jersey Medical Reporter* 5, no. 10 (1852), 371–372.

GIVE THAT MAN A MEDAL

W. M. Chamberlain, "Remarkable recovery from gunshot, sabre, bayonet, and shell wounds," *Medical Record* 10 (1875), 685.

"The courts: Making a false pension claim," *New York Daily Herald*, March 6, 1867, 4.

"Personated a dead man," *Brooklyn Daily Eagle*, June 22, 1890, 18.

A BIT OF A HEADACHE

"Singulier cas de suicide: un poignard dans le crâne produisant une plaie de cerveau sans symptômes," *Journal de Médecine et de Chirurgie Pratiques* 52 (1881), 366–367.

6. TALL TALES

Alexander Munro (primus), "The preface," *Medical Essays and Observations* 1 (1733), i-xxiv.

William Pickells, "Case of a young woman, who has discharged, and continues to discharge, from her stomach, a number of insects, in different stages of their existence," *Transactions of the Association of Fellows and Licentiates of the King and Queen's College of Physicians in Ireland* 4 (1824), 189–221.

SLEEPING WITH THE FISHES

Rowland Jackson, *A Physical Dissertation on Drowning* (London: Jacob Robinson, 1746), 10–16.

DEATH OF A 152-YEAR-OLD

John Taylor, *The Old, Old, Very Old Man* (London: Henry Goffon, 1635).

Robert Willis (ed.), *The Works of William Harvey* (London: Sydenham Society, 1847), 589–592.

Keith Thomas, "Parr, Thomas," *Oxford Dictionary of National Biography,* https://doi.org/10.1093/ref:odnb/21403.

THE COMBUSTIBLE COUNTESS

Paul Rolli, "An extract, by Mr. Paul Rolli FRS of an Italian treatise, written by the Reverend Joseph Bianchini, a prebend in the city of Verona; upon the death of the countess Cornelia Zangári & Bandi, of Ceséna. To which are subjoined accounts of the death of Jo. Hitchell, who was burned to death by lightning; and of Grace Pett at Ipswich, whose body was consumed to a Coal," *Philosophical Transactions* 43, no. 476 (1744), 447–465.

HE SLICED HIS PENIS IN TWO

François Chopart, *Traité des Maladies des Voies Urinaires* (2 vols; Paris: Rémont et fils, 1821), 2: 114–118, translated in Alfred Poulet, *A Treatise on Foreign Bodies in Surgical Practice* (2 vols; London: Sampson Low, Marston, Searle & Rivington, 1881), 2: 105–107.

HALF MAN, HALF SNAKE

"Robert H. Copeland," *Southern Medical and Surgical Journal* 3, no. 6 (1839), 381–382.

THE HUMAN WAXWORK

"Extraordinary case of adipocere," *Western Medical Reformer* 6, no. 11 (1847), 238.

"Human fat candles and soap," *Scientific American* 8, no. 7 (1852), 56.

THE SLUGS AND THE PORCUPINE

David Dickman, "Can the garden slug live in the human stomach?" *Lancet* 74, no. 1883 (1859), 337.

J. C. Dalton, "Experimental investigations to determine whether the garden slug can live in the human stomach," *American Journal of the Medical Sciences* 49, no. 97 (1865), 334–338.

THE AMPHIBIOUS INFANT

"Fish, frog or human!," *Northern Ohio Journal* 2, no 39 (April 2, 1873), 1.

"An amphibious infant," *Medical Notes and Queries* 1, no. 1 (1873), 7.

THE SEVENTY-YEAR-OLD MOTHER-TO-BE

"Variétés," *Journal de Médecine de Paris* 1, no. 26 (1881), 715.

7. HIDDEN DANGERS

"Impaired voice, in clergymen," *Boston Medical and Surgical Journal* 20, no. 7 (1839), 112–113.

A SURFEIT OF CUCUMBERS

William Perfect, "Appearances on opening the body of a woman, who died the beginning of August 1762, after eating a large quantity of cucumbers," *Medical Museum* 1 (1781), 212–213.

THE PERILS OF BEING A WRITER

J. S. Jenkins, "Dr. Samuel Auguste Tissot," *Journal of Medical Biography* 7, no. 4 (1999), 187–191.

Samuel Auguste David Tissot, *An Essay on Diseases Incident to Literary and Sedentary Persons* (London: J. Nourse, 1769).

WHY CHILDREN SHOULD NEVER WEAR HATS

Bernhard Christoph Faust (trans. J. H. Basse), *Catechism of Health, for the Use of Schools, and for Domestic Instruction* (London: C. Dilly, 1794), 37–46.

KILLED BY HIS FALSE TEETH

W. G. Carpenter, "Case of fatal pleuritis, apparently the effect of the presence in
the right pleura of a piece of ivory, consisting of four artificial teeth, which had
been swallowed thirteen years before," *Guy's Hospital Reports* 7 (1842),
353–358.

PEGGED OUT

Robert B. Carter, "Cases in practice," *Ophthalmic Review* 1 (1865), 335–343.

THE CAST-IRON STOVE PANIC

"Medical annotations," *Lancet* 91, no. 2324 (1868), 354–358.

A. J. Morin, "Mémoire sur l'insalubrité des poêles en fonte ou en fer exposés à
atteindre la température rouge," *Mémoires de l'Académie des Sciences de
l'Institut de France* 38 (1873), 23–90.

BROLLY PAINFUL

"Transactions of societies," *Medical Press and Circular* 15 (1873), 249–259.

A FLAMING NUISANCE

"Clinical memoranda," *British Medical Journal* 1, no. 1311 (1886), 294–296.

R. Scott Orr, "Cases of inflammable expired air," *British Medical Journal* 1, no.
1313 (1886), 421.

James McNaught, "A case of dilatation of the stomach accompanied by the
eructation of inflammable gas," *British Medical Journal* 1, no. 1522 (1890),
470–472.

Archibald H. Galley, "Combustible gases generated in the alimentary tract and
other hollow viscera and their relationship to explosions occurring during
anaesthesia," *British Journal of Anaesthesia* 26, no. 3 (1954), 189–193.

CYCLING WILL GIVE YOU HEART DISEASE

George Herschell, "On cycling as a cause of heart disease," in Zsigmond Gerlóczy
(ed.), *Jelentés az 1894. Szeptember hó 1-töl 9-ig Budapesten Tartott VIII-ik
Nemzetközi Közegészségi és Demografiai Congressusról és Annak Tudományos
Munkálatairól* (Vol 6; Budapest: Pesti Könyvnyomda-Részvénytársaság, 1896),
9–17.

ACKNOWLEDGMENTS

Grateful thanks to Stephen Morrow at Dutton for his astute and careful work on the manuscript, which turned this labor into a pleasure. And to my agent, Patrick Walsh, whose enthusiasm and energy got the project off the ground. Rohin Francis, Andrea Sella, Hugh Devlin, and Stéphane Burtey offered obscure diagnoses and other specialist expertise, which was much appreciated—as did my wife, Jenny, who endures my queries with heroic forbearance. Thanks to all of you.

INDEX

---

* I'll be honest, there's a lot of blood in this book. If that's what you're after, you can hardly miss it.

About the Author

Thomas Morris is a writer and medical historian. His first book, *The Matter of the Heart*, a history of heart surgery, was a winner of a Royal Society of Literature Jerwood Award. He lives in London.